MUSIC THERAPY AND GERIATRIC POPULATIONS:

A Handbook for Practicing Music Therapists and Healthcare Professionals

MUSIC THERAPY AND GERIATRIC POPULATIONS:

A Handbook for Practicing Music Therapists and Healthcare Professionals

Melita Belgrave, PhD, MT-BC
Alice-Ann Darrow, PhD, MT-BC
Darcy Walworth, PhD, MT-BC
Natalie Wlodarczyk, PhD, MT-BC

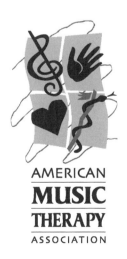

AMERICAN
MUSIC
THERAPY
ASSOCIATION

The American Music Therapy Association is a non-profit association dedicated to increasing access to quality music therapy services for individuals with disabilities or illnesses or for those who are interested in personal growth and wellness. AMTA provides extensive educational and research information about the music therapy profession. Referrals for qualified music therapists are also provided to consumers and parents. AMTA holds an annual conference every autumn and its seven regions hold conferences every spring.

For up-to-date information, please access the AMTA website at www.musictherapy.org

ISBN: **978-1-884914-28-7**

Copyright Information: **© by American Music Therapy Association, Inc., 2011**
8455 Colesville Road, Suite 1000
Silver Spring, Maryland 20910 USA
www.musictherapy.org
info@musictherapy.org

Technical Assistance: **Wordsetters**
Kalamazoo, Michigan

Cover Design: **Tawna Grasty/Grass T Design**

Printed in the United States of America

ACKNOWLEDGMENTS

This work was supported by HRSA Geriatrics Education Center grant No. D13HP08843 and The Florida State University College of Medicine and College of Music

A special thanks to Ken Brummel-Smith, MD, and Alice Pomidor, MD

CONTENTS

Music therapy is a non-invasive treatment strategy that can be useful in the clinical work of healthcare professionals who service geriatric populations. Music therapy interventions have long been used to address the physical, emotional, social, and cognitive needs of older persons. With the rapid growth of the aging population and the increasing number of persons who are diagnosed each year with age-related disorders, music therapists and healthcare workers need to be familiar with the ways in which music can be used to enhance the plan of care for aging adults.

The purpose of this handbook is to provide information to music therapists and to healthcare professionals on the uses of music therapy with four common geriatric populations:

1. Adults with Alzheimer's disease
2. Adults in hospice care
3. Adults in health and wellness programs
4. Adults in intergenerational programs

Music therapists are academically and clinically trained in the uses of music to address the needs of older persons. The clinical and musical expertise of a board-certified music therapist is always preferable. Other healthcare professionals, however, may wish to use music therapy in providing care to aging adults in hospitals and assisted living or nursing facilities. Music therapists typically work during the daytime hours, and there are frequently times during the evening or weekends when healthcare workers may find music interventions useful for clients, especially those who may be experiencing pain or stress.

The focus of the handbook is threefold:

1. To educate music therapists and healthcare professionals about the uses and evidence-based benefits of music therapy practices with older adults;
2. To familiarize music therapists and healthcare professionals with clinical applications trained music therapists can provide to older adults;
3. To present selected ways healthcare professionals—both with and without musical training—can use music in their work with older adults.

For each of the adult populations, the handbook includes three chapters. The first chapter provides practical introductory information on the specific adult population. The second chapter is a review of related music therapy research. This research review provides the basis for the third chapter—clinical applications of evidence-based music therapy practice. The final chapter in each unit includes a hierarchical ordering of the clinical applications. The applications are successively structured for (a) general staff or volunteers with no musical training, (b) general staff or volunteers with some musical training or music skills, and (c) board-certified music therapists who have advanced skills in music and working with older adults. With these applications for music therapists and other health-related professions, music can become an integral part of the comprehensive care plan for adult clients.

What is music therapy?

Music therapy is the clinical and evidence-based use of music interventions to accomplish individualized goals within a therapeutic relationship by a credentialed professional who has completed an approved music therapy program (American Music Therapy Association website, 2011).

What do music therapists do?

Music therapists assess emotional well-being, physical health, social functioning, communication abilities, and cognitive skills through musical responses; design music sessions for individuals and groups based on client needs using music improvisation, receptive music listening, songwriting, lyric discussion, music and imagery, music performance, and learning through music; and participate in interdisciplinary treatment planning, ongoing evaluation, and follow up.

Who can benefit from music therapy?

Children, adolescents, adults, and the elderly with mental health needs, developmental and learning disabilities, Alzheimer's disease and other aging-related conditions, substance abuse problems, brain injuries, physical disabilities, and acute and chronic pain, including mothers in labor.

Where do music therapists work?

Music therapists work in psychiatric hospitals, rehabilitative facilities, medical hospitals, outpatient clinics, daycare treatment centers, agencies serving persons with developmental disabilities, community mental health centers, drug and alcohol programs, senior centers, nursing homes, hospice programs, correctional facilities, halfway houses, schools, and private practice.

What is the history of music therapy as a health care profession?

The idea of music as a healing influence that could affect health and behavior is as least as old as the writings of Aristotle and Plato. The 20th century discipline began after World War I and World War II when community musicians of all types, both amateur and professional, went to veterans hospitals around the country to play for the thousands of veterans suffering both physical and emotional trauma from the wars. The patients' notable physical and emotional responses to music led the doctors and nurses to request the hiring of musicians by the hospitals. It was soon evident that the hospital musicians needed some prior training before entering the facility, and so the demand grew for a college curriculum. The first music therapy degree program in the world, founded at Michigan State University in 1944, celebrated its 50th anniversary in 1994. The American Music Therapy Association was founded in 1998 as a union of the National Association for Music Therapy and the American Association for Music Therapy.

Who is qualified to practice music therapy?

Persons who complete one of the approved college music therapy curricula (including an internship) are then eligible to sit for the national examination offered by the Certification Board for Music Therapists. Music therapists who successfully complete the independently administered examination hold the music therapist-board certified credential (MT-BC).

The National Music Therapy Registry (NMTR) serves qualified music therapy professionals with the following designations: RMT, CMT, ACMT. These individuals have met accepted educational and clinical training standards and are qualified to practice music therapy.

Is there research to support music therapy?

AMTA promotes a vast amount of research exploring the benefits of music as therapy through publication of the *Journal of Music Therapy*, *Music Therapy Perspectives*, and other sources. A substantial body of literature exists to support the effectiveness of music therapy.

What are some misconceptions about music therapy?

That the client or patient has to have some particular music ability to benefit from music therapy—they do not. That there is one particular style of music that is more therapeutic than all the rest—this is not the case. All styles of music can be useful in effecting change in a client or patient's life. The individual's preferences, circumstances, and need for treatment, and the client or patient's goals help to determine the types of music a music therapist may use.

How can music therapy techniques be applied by healthy individuals?

Healthy individuals can use music for stress reduction via active music making, such as drumming, as well as passive listening for relaxation. Music is often a vital support for physical exercise. Music therapy assisted labor and delivery may also be included in this category since pregnancy is regarded as a normal part of women's life cycles.

How is music therapy utilized in hospitals?

Music is used in general hospitals to alleviate pain in conjunction with anesthesia or pain medication; elevate patients' mood and counteract depression; promote movement for physical rehabilitation; calm or sedate, often to induce sleep; counteract apprehension or fear; and lessen muscle tension for the purpose of relaxation, including the autonomic nervous system.

How is music therapy utilized in nursing homes?

Music is used with elderly persons to increase or maintain their level of physical, mental, and social/emotional functioning. The sensory and intellectual stimulation of music can help maintain a person's quality of life.

Is music therapy a reimbursable service?

- *Medicare*

  - *Partial Hospitalization Programs (PHP)*

    Since 1994, music therapy has been identified as a reimbursable service under the benefits for Partial Hospitalization Programs (PHP). Under the heading of Activity Therapy, using the HCPCS code G0176, music therapy must be considered an active treatment by meeting the following criteria:

    - Physician's prescription;
    - Reasonable and necessary for the treatment of the individual's illness or injury; and
    - Goal directed and based on a documented treatment plan.

  - *Prospective Payment System (PPS)*

    Under Medicare's Prospective Payment System (PPS) music therapy is not billed as a separate service, but can be included as part of the treatment team within skilled nursing facilities/nursing homes, in-patient psychiatric programs, hospice programs, and in-patient rehab settings. Music therapists contribute to a facility's treatment program and are included within the PPS daily reimbursement, assisting the facility to implement cost-effective services.

  - *Minimum Data Set (MDS)*

    The MDS assessment tool utilized in skilled nursing facilities and some residential care centers has many sections in which music therapists can provide input to the treatment team, but not all sections of this document have an impact on the reimbursement a facility receives from Medicare. To assist facilities access additional funding, music therapists can document minutes under Restorative Care. Several programs that music therapists typically provide in skilled or residential care facilities may fall under Restorative Care. Exercise programs, socialization groups, and orientation sessions are a few examples of interventions that might help to address Restorative Care needs of clients. The best way to explore this option of documenting music therapy under the Restorative Care section of the MDS is by collaborating with the MDS coordinator in a facility.

    The MDS 3.0 assessment tool also lists music therapy under Section O. Special Treatments and Procedures, O0400. Therapies, F. Recreational Therapy (includes recreational and music therapy). Although this listing does not provide additional reimbursement for the facility, it does provide a more accurate vehicle for documenting physician-ordered music therapy services in settings utilizing the MDS and helps to validate the inclusion of music therapy as a part of the PPS daily rate.

- *Medicaid Waivers*

  Medicaid waivers are programs developed by each state that focus on specific client groups or diagnoses and provide additional services that are not covered by other funding sources. There are currently a few states that allow payment for music therapy services through use of Medicaid Home and Community Based Care waivers with certain client groups. In some situations, although music therapy may not be specifically listed within regulatory language, due to functional outcomes achieved, music therapy interventions qualify for coverage under existing treatment categories such as community support, rehabilitation, or habilitation services

- *Private Insurance*

The number of success stories involving private insurance reimbursement for the provision of music therapy services continues to grow. Companies like Blue Cross Blue Shield, United Healthcare, Cigna, and Aetna and others have all reimbursed for music therapy services at some time on a case-by-case basis. Success has occurred when the therapist implements steps within the reimbursement process and receives pre-approval for music therapy services.

Communicating with case managers, music therapists provide required documentation for insurance industry representatives to make informed decisions about music therapy coverage. Board Certified Music Therapists record assessment results, propose treatment plans, outline functional outcomes of music therapy interventions, provide diagnostic and procedure codes, and present research evidence to support the reimbursement process. Music therapy can be a reimbursable service when deemed medically or behaviorally necessary to attain the treatment goals of the individual client.

- *Other Sources*

Additional sources for reimbursement and financing of music therapy services include: state and county departments of mental health, state and county departments of developmental disabilities, workers' compensation, private auto insurance, Individuals with Disabilities Education Act Part B funding, foundations, grants, and private pay.

What is the American Music Therapy Association?

The American Music Therapy Association (AMTA) represents over 5,000 music therapists, corporate members, and related associations worldwide. AMTA's roots date back to organizations founded in 1950 and 1971. Those two organizations merged in 1998 to ensure the progressive development of the therapeutic use of music in rehabilitation, special education, and medical and community settings. AMTA is committed to the advancement of education, training, professional standards, and research in support of the music therapy profession. The mission of the organization is to advance public knowledge of music therapy benefits and increase access to quality music therapy services. Currently, AMTA establishes criteria for the education and clinical training of music therapists. Members of AMTA adhere to a Code of Ethics and Standards of Practice in their delivery of music therapy services.

Source: Copyright © 2011, American Music Therapy Association

DEFINITIONS OF MUSIC THERAPY INTERVENTIONS USED WITH GERIATRIC POPULATIONS

Music Therapy Intervention	Definition	Application
Gait Training with Music	MT-BC uses an auditory cue to improve aspects of a patient's gait such as cadence, velocity, and overall cycle. Rhythm and speed of auditory cue is matched to patient's current gait speed and then gradually increased to desired speed. Auditory cues are presented as a metronome beat, drum beat, or recorded instrumental music.	• Improve gait cadence • Improve gait velocity • Improve overall gait cycle
Imagery with Music	MT-BC guides patient through imagery exercises with instrumental music. MT-BC directs patients to imagine a place or setting that is soothing and comfortable to them.	• Decrease pain perception • Decrease anxiety • Increase relaxation
Instrument Play	MT-BC provides patient with a variety of instruments to play. Instruments are chosen so that patient can be successful without musical training. Instrument play interventions include unstructured playing, playing in rhythm, and specific rhythmic patterns.	• Provide opportunity for self-expression • Facilitate use of short-term memory • Maintain attention • Increase range of motion • Provide opportunity for physical activity
Iso-Principle	The use of music to change patient affect or behaviors. MT-BC matches the volume of voice and accompaniment instrument to patient-exhibited behavior. MT-BC then changes volume of voice, accompaniment instrument, and accompaniment style to change patient behavior.	• Decrease pain perception • Decrease agitation • Increase relaxation
Life Review with Music or Music Cued Reminiscence	MT-BC uses music as a structure and cue for recalling and processing important events in a patient's life. Life review occurs in an individual session, whereas music cued reminiscence occurs in a group setting.	• Provide opportunity for reflection • Provide opportunity for closure at end-of-life • Enhance mood through recall of pleasant memories

Music Therapy Intervention	Definition	Application
Living Legacy Project	MT-BC assists patient to create product of special memories to leave for family. Products usually include: CD recordings of the patient and music therapist singing songs that were special to the family, scrapbooks with pictures, stories and special song lyrics, or video projects.	▪ Provide a lasting product that the family can keep ▪ Aid in bereavement for the family after the patient's death
Movement to Music	MT-BC pairs physical movements with music to provide both structure and motivation for patients to participate. Movements range from specific motions to a chosen song, to free movement that is patient-led.	▪ Increase physical exercise ▪ Increase wellness ▪ Increase self-expression ▪ Increase range of motion
Music Listening	MT-BC leads patient in active music listening. MT-BC gives patient a task to complete that corresponds to changes in the music.	▪ Maintain attention ▪ Increase orientation to environment ▪ Facilitate use of aural discrimination skills
Progressive Muscle Relaxation with Music	MT-BC leads exercises that result in a succession of tightening and releasing of muscle groups in the body. The relaxation series is completed in rhythm to instrumental music. Instrumental music is sedative and is presented either live or recorded.	▪ Decrease pain perception ▪ Decrease agitation ▪ Decrease anxiety ▪ Increase relaxation
Sensory Stimulation with Music	MT-BC provides opportunity for patient visual and tactile stimulation through singing and playing instruments.	▪ Increase orientation to environment ▪ Maintain attention
Songwriting	MT-BC assists patient in writing lyrics to a song. Lyrics to songs can be original or adapted from a familiar song.	▪ Provides opportunity for self-expression
Therapeutic Singing	MT-BC sings patient-preferred music to structure session. Patient sings along, if able.	▪ Improve orientation to environment ▪ Enhance interactions

UNIT I
MUSIC THERAPY AND PERSONS WITH ALZHEIMER'S DISEASE

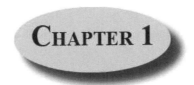

INTRODUCTION TO ALZHEIMER'S DISEASE
AND MUSIC THERAPY

Oohh . . . I used to dance to that song at every dance with my husband! I just love hearing your music. —Mrs. S.

I like picking up Momma on the days when you are here. She is so calm when you play for her. —Mrs. D.

As a person ages, it is common to experience a decline in cognitive functioning. Not all cognitive decline results in dementia related disorders; therefore, it is important for healthcare professionals to know the differences in presenting symptoms so that appropriate evaluation referrals can be made. Mild cognitive decline, such as difficulty naming objects, changes in immediate memory, and declines in visual and verbal memory, may be attributed to the normal aging process; however, a person's vocabulary and verbal reasoning do not typically change throughout the normal aging process.

Symptoms of dementia differ from those that occur due to the normal aging process. Differences are in frequency of symptom occurrences, as well as in social functioning or independent living. When an individual experiences multiple cognitive deficits in areas such as spatial, working, and verbal memory, executive functioning, and use of language, symptoms should be observed and a referral made for evaluation. Typical symptoms shown by individuals suffering from dementia include asking the same questions multiple times, exhibiting changes in personality and eating habits, paying less attention to hygiene, getting lost in areas that were previously familiar, having difficulty comprehending spoken language, showing lack of motivation, losing balance more easily, and exhibiting behaviors that seem odd or inappropriate (Gazzaley, 2009). The most common forms of dementia and their characteristics are:

- Mixed dementia—most commonly seen with hallmark features of Alzheimer's disease occurring with symptoms of vascular dementia, although any two forms of dementia constitute this type of dementia. Current studies are suggesting mixed dementia is more common than thought in the past.
- Parkinson's disease—dementia symptoms typically show during the late stage of Parkinson's disease and are attributed to Lewy bodies forming inside nerve cells of the brain.
- Creutzfeldt-Jakob disease—occurs for individuals who ingest foods from cattle with mad cow disease, when the brain experiences misfolding of prion proteins. This disorder is fatal and includes a rapid decline in memory, coordination, and marked behavior changes.

- Alzheimer's disease—the most common form of dementia accounting for up to 80% of all dementia cases. Clinical abnormalities include plaques consisting of deposits of the protein fragment beta-amyloid and tangles made of twisted strands of the protein tau (Alzheimer's Association, 2010).

To be diagnosed with dementia, a person must have deficits severe enough to interfere with the ability to function in his or her daily life, show a decline in memory functioning, and show decline in at least one of the following cognition functions:

1. ability to generate coherent speech or understand spoken or written language;
2. ability to recognize or identify objects, assuming intact sensory function;
3. ability to execute motor activities, assuming intact motor abilities, sensory function, and comprehension of the required task;
4. ability to think abstractly, make sound judgments, and plan and carry out complex tasks (Alzheimer's Association, 2010).

ALZHEIMER'S DISEASE

Alzheimer's disease affects the brain's ability to transfer information at the synapses, with the number of synapses declining over time and, eventually, brain cells dying (Alzheimer's Association, 2010). Researchers over the last 30 years have focused on the behavioral and lifestyle differences between people with normal age-related cognitive declines, dementia, and Alzheimer's disease as well as effective symptom management (Derwinger, Stigsdotter Neely, MacDonald, & Backman, 2005; O'Hara et al., 2007; Willis et al., 2006). Their findings have led to current research investigating genetic factors in combination with biological and environmental factors that affect the progression of Alzheimer's disease and address the underlying issues of the disease. Alzheimer's disease is now understood to have genetic links with genetic variants possibly leading to a genetic risk factor for being diagnosed with the disease (Alzheimer's Disease Education and Referral Center [ADEAR], 2008a, 2010). People who are later diagnosed with Alzheimer's disease generally show symptoms after the age of 60. While not all people with dementia will later be diagnosed with Alzheimer's disease, it is the leading cause of dementia for elderly adults, affecting as many as 5.1 million Americans. This irreversible brain disease will eventually result in impairing an individual's ability to carry out even simple tasks. Group and individualized interventions that have been investigated to address slowing down the cognitive decline include cognitive training programs, memory training, cognitive stimulation to increase cognitive and social functioning, cognitive rehabilitation programs, physical exercise, music interventions, activity groups, support groups, counseling, and adult day center programs (Alzheimer's Association, 2010; Clair, 1996; Clair, Mathews, & Kosloski, 2005; Hampstead, Sathian, Moore, Nalisnick, & Stringer, 2008; Jean, Bergeron, Thivierge, & Simard, 2010; Kinsella et al., 2009; Mariani, Monastero, & Mecocci, 2007; Troyer, Murphy, Anderson, Moscovitch, & Craik, 2008).

Diagnosing Alzheimer's Disease

The diagnosis of Alzheimer's disease cannot be made until after death, when an autopsy is conducted. However, physicians are able to give a probable Alzheimer's disease diagnosis based on various cognitive tests, combined with behavioral signs, family and individual history, blood and spinal fluid tests, and radiology scans such as Computerized Tomography or Magnetic Resonance Imaging (ADEAR, 2010). Many tests are used to evaluate cognitive function. The most common is the Mini-Mental State Examination, but additional helpful information can be obtained from tests including Logical Memory, East Boston Story, Word List Memory, Word List Recognition, Boston Naming Test, Verbal Fluency, Digit Span Forward, Digit Span Backward, Digit Ordering, Symbol Digit Modalities Test, Number Comparison, Stroop Neuropsychological Screening Test, Judgment of Line Orientation, and Standard Progressive Matrices (Boyle, Buchman, Barnes, & Bennett, 2010). Generally, when an individual exhibits a decline in behavioral skills and self-care, in addition to cognitive impairment, a probable Alzheimer's disease diagnosis can be made.

Due to advances in diagnostic tools, many people who receive early-stage diagnosis are aware and can comprehend exactly what their diagnosis of Alzheimer's disease means to themselves and their family members. The result can be feelings of embarrassment, isolation, depressed mood, and sometimes denial. It is recommended that individuals and families who have accepted the reality of the diagnosis be involved in early-stage support groups to foster a sense of community, mental stimulation, and education about the stressors and planning needs for the future. The emotional support, networking, sense of control, and preparedness for upcoming struggles have been reported as beneficial and helpful for families and individuals with an early-stage diagnosis (ADEAR, 2009).

Prevalence of Alzheimer's Disease

In studies investigating prevalence rates for men versus women, the finding that more women than men have dementia and Alzheimer's disease has been attributed to women living longer lives than men (Alzheimer's Association, 2010). There do not seem to be any correlations between females being at higher risk for developing Alzheimer's disease or dementia. Because women tend to live longer, the data reflect that women are more affected than men, with 16% of women and 11% of men receiving a dementia diagnosis. Recent investigations of prevalence rates by race for Alzheimer's disease and other dementias have indicated that African Americans are twice as likely as older Caucasians to have Alzheimer's and other dementias (Alzheimer's Association, 2010). This information is helpful for professionals planning interventions for the demographic area they serve.

Etiology of Alzheimer's Disease

The cause of Alzheimer's disease is still unknown, and there is still no cure or way to prevent onset of the disease. There are common age-related features of the brain that possibly contribute to the damage seen in people with Alzheimer's disease, including shrinking of the brain, free radicals, and inflammation of the brain. Studies are continuing to look into the three hallmark features of Alzheimer's disease: plaques, neurofibrillary tangles, and loss of connections between cells and cell death in the brain of individuals affected by Alzheimer's disease. Brain imaging now allows researchers to see plaques forming in the brain while people are still alive. This could lead to the ability to establish early diagnosis procedures with corresponding early treatment. The plaques that form in the brain first appear in the neocortex, and later spread throughout the brain. Similarly, the neurofibrillary tangles that originally affect a small area of the brain will eventually affect a very large area (Alzheimer's Association, 2010). When neurons are affected to the point they can no longer function, they can die off, causing brain atrophy and brain tissue shrinkage seen in autopsies of individuals with Alzheimer's disease (ADEAR, 2008b).

Amyloid plaques are located between the brain's nerve cells and are made up of an insoluble toxic protein peptide called beta-amyloid. It is still unknown if the amyloid plaques cause Alzheimer's disease, or if the progression of Alzheimer's disease causes the plaques to form and spread. In the past, it was commonly believed that the plaques actually caused the neuron damage seen in the brain of individuals with Alzheimer's disease. More recent research has pointed to the formation of the plaques to try to protect neurons in the brain from the debilitating beta-amyloid. The major agent causing the damage is now thought to be oligomers, which are made up of 2 to 12 soluble aggregates of beta-amyloid peptides (ADEAR, 2008a).

The *tau* protein is the primary component of the brain forming neurofibrillary tangles. These are identified by looking inside nerve cells and finding abnormal collections of twisted protein threads. Hyperphosphorylation results in an abnormally large number of phosphate molecules that attach to tau, causing the tau to disengage from its normal attachment to microtubules. The resulting attachment to other tau strands leads to the formation of neurofibrillary tangles. An important function of neuron communication is then lost as the damaged microtubules disintegrate (ADEAR, 2008a).

Categorization of Alzheimer's Disease

Previously described as early-, middle-, and late-stage Alzheimer's, researchers now categorize the disease by severity. The progression starts with very early Alzheimer's, leading to mild Alzheimer's, followed by moderate, and, finally, severe Alzheimer's disease. Most often, people are diagnosed in the mild Alzheimer's stage, as they exhibit mood and personality changes, memory difficulties when performing tasks such as paying bills, and poor judgment when attempting to make decisions. As the disease progresses to moderate Alzheimer's, damage can be seen in the brain in areas that control sensory processing, language, reasoning, and conscious thought (ADEAR, 2010). At this stage, it may be difficult for a person with Alzheimer's disease to recognize family members and friends. Additionally, the individual may experience difficulty in completing, without assistance, tasks that require multiple steps, such as getting dressed. Hallucinations may begin to occur, along with paranoia, delusions, and impulsive behaviors. Severe Alzheimer's disease is characterized by individuals spending most or all of the day in bed with complete dependence on others for care. Also, at this stage, people experience an inability to communicate, as the body shuts down (ADEAR, 2008b).

The results of many studies are used to inform and determine the most effective way to manage the disease for individuals and their loved ones. Maintaining the highest possible level of functioning is the ultimate goal for clinicians and medical staff involved in caring for an individual affected by Alzheimer's. To do so effectively, long-term monitoring of symptoms is required. Because Alzheimer's is a degenerative disease, caregivers require long-term support to address the newest challenges presented as their loved one is faced with increasing impairments.

Caregivers' Emotions and Needs

Caring for an individual with Alzheimer's disease is a process that affects the emotional, physical, financial, and social areas of a caregiver's life. Agencies such as the National Institute on Aging, the Alzheimer's Association, and Alzheimer's Disease Centers have focused on the needs of the caregiver. Education, support, and resources are imperative for those who provide care to an individual affected by Alzheimer's disease. The multi-faceted struggles that caregivers face can be alleviated through various means, including support groups, educational training, complementary therapies and interventions, and wellness centers focusing on the whole health of individuals.

Caregivers can experience different stages of emotional adjustment following their loved one's diagnosis (Austrom & Lu, 2009; Kaplan, 1996). When a caregiver is in denial, the loved one's problems are often excused as something other than a decline in cognitive functioning. Conversely, a caregiver who is aware of the problems faced by a loved one may become overinvolved and compensate, in an unhealthy way, for the deficits displayed by the individual with Alzheimer's. Anger is another emotional adjustment issue commonly seen in caregivers, resulting from the many different struggles in caring for a loved one. Some feel angry because they are unable to alter the course of the progressing disease. Others experience anger because of embarrassing situations their loved ones create due to forgetfulness, outbursts, or personality changes. Some caregivers may displace their anger, directing it toward family members, even though they have not personally angered the caregiver. Caregiver burdens commonly cause anger when caregiving is the primary responsibility of one individual and is not shared by other family members. Such anger can also lead to feelings of guilt, or, when suppressed, can result in depression for the caregiver. Guilt can also stem from feelings of failure when caregivers are unable to meet their loved one's needs as the disease progresses. Most caregivers eventually accept the individual's diagnosis, which inevitably leads to a grieving process over the loss of the loved one they once knew.

Additional issues facing caregivers can be clustered in the following areas (Austrom & Lu, 2009; Dhooper, 1991; Kaplan, 1996):

- *Family disruptions* can occur when family members change roles, experience an overload in familial roles, and have conflicts within the family due to the diagnosis.
- *Psychological stress* is experienced when there is depression about the circumstances, self-blame for their loved one's behaviors, anger and resentment of the disease's progression, loneliness from increased caregiving demands, and deterioration of the patient.
- *Physical fatigue* occurs as the disease progresses over time and the demands continue and/or increase for the caregiver.
- *Social isolation* results from avoidance of social situations with friends and family members due to embarrassing behaviors exhibited by the individual as the disease progresses, as well as decreased time and energy to engage in social situations due to increased caregiving demands.
- *Financial issues* result from decreased income of the patient or caregiver, increased feelings of anxiety about impending costs associated with long-term care of the patient, and medical expenses associated with the disease over time.
- *Legal issues* arise due to the patient's decreasing mental competence as the disease progresses.

Individualizing support services and care for the caregiver is recommended. Caregivers experience shifts in their emotional and support needs over time, necessitating varying levels of involvement from healthcare professionals and support staff. Although group interventions are appropriate and helpful, individualized sessions allow the interventions to be targeted to the most relevant needs a caregiver is facing. Intervention techniques that address all of the issues caregivers face are recommended due to the fluctuating responses caregivers can exhibit during the care process (Austrom & Lu, 2009).

MUSIC THERAPY AND ALZHEIMER'S DISEASE

Music therapy has become an accepted, research-based treatment for individuals at all stages of Alzheimer's disease. Music plays a prominent role in most people's lives and is an important component of memories of weddings, dances, dates, concerts attended, and home life. Listening to specific songs can stimulate such memories and reminiscence. Music therapists are trained to use music that is meaningful to each patient to address specific needs. As a result, music therapy has been used to achieve goals such as orientation to time and place; maintenance of social behaviors; reduction of anxiety, agitation, and restlessness; maintenance of receptive and expressive language skills; reduction of disruptive behaviors; maintenance of memory functions; increased positive affect; and improved caregiver relationships (Brotons, 2003; Carruth, 1997; Clair, 1996; Clair & Bernstein, 1990; Gerdner, 1999; Hanson, Gfeller, Woodworth, Swanson, & Garand, 1996; Koger, Chapin, & Brotons; 1999; Smith, 1986). Music therapy can greatly contribute to the overall highest level of patient-centered care. The music therapist, with the rest of the care team, works to identify specific goals, assess progress, and implement appropriate interventions for each patient. Music therapists can elicit desired patient behaviors due to the interactive and stimulating qualities inherent in music.

Music therapy interventions can be implemented in an individual session or in a group setting. Some of the interventions employed in music therapy sessions include reminiscence, movement to music, instrument playing, singing, songwriting, and memory training. While some of these activities can be led by volunteers or other staff, music therapists are specifically trained to assess patient needs while patients are engaged in activities. This type of ongoing assessment maximizes the benefits of the music therapy intervention for patients. An additional benefit of working with a board-certified music therapist is the resulting patient-centered care provided. The structure and content of each music therapy session is customized to fit the constantly changing status of the patient, resulting in highly individualized care. The individualization within each music therapy session is largely a result of song choices by each patient—one song may elicit a different response across patients within a group. A song that elicits pleasant and happy memories for one patient may evoke feelings of sadness and loss for another patient. The specialized training in counseling that music therapists receive enables them to address each patient's feelings and needs, even when contrasting patient responses are exhibited simultaneously.

Research has investigated music therapy interventions for maintaining skills across domains of persons who are in the early to middle stages of dementia. Researched goals have included increasing active participation in groups and social behaviors, decreasing disruptive behaviors and depressive symptoms, and improving language functioning (Brotons & Pickett-Cooper, 1996; Cevasco & Grant, 2003; Clair & Bernstein, 1990; Clair et al., 2005; Hanson et al., 1996; Olderog-Millard & Smith, 1989; Pollack & Namazi, 1992). The use of live music in activities elicited greater arousal and socialization from individuals with dementia than when recorded music was used (O'Connor, Ames, Gardner, & King,

2009). Movement activities were most effective in engaging individuals with dementia in purposeful participation, and participants were more purposefully involved in rhythm and singing activities when those activities were presented at lower levels of demand (Hanson et al., 1996). Also, group participation tended to increase during movement exercises when recorded instrumental music was used and the music therapist gave a continuous verbal cue following the rhythmic structure of the piece of music (Cevasco & Grant, 2003).

Staff members can be involved and can be taught how to lead activities using music. Activity staff with little to no formal music training who were employed by a facility treating patients with mid-stage dementia were taught by a music therapist to use a music protocol that included rhythm playing, exercising with music, and singing. The protocol was accessible and successful for the staff members. Individuals with dementia participated consistently over time and across each of the three music activities. While only a board-certified music therapist can provide music therapy and best-practice, this protocol provides an alternative for facilities in areas where music therapists are unavailable.

Live music therapy interventions can decrease agitation levels of persons with dementia both during a music therapy session and for a period of time after the session ends (Brotons & Pickett-Cooper, 1996; Raglio et al., 2008). Individuals with dementia exhibit less agitation when their individually preferred music is played as compared to generally selected recorded music (O'Connor et al., 2009). Since displays of agitation can hinder positive connection during family visits, scheduling music therapy sessions before common visiting times is beneficial for both patients and family members. Music therapy can also have a lasting positive effect on delusions, anxiety, apathy, irritability, aberrant motor activity, and nighttime behavior disturbances (Raglio et al., 2008).

Many facilities have discussion sessions to foster socialization and communication for patients with dementia. When comparing music therapy sessions to non-music discussion sessions, patients exhibit significantly higher vocal/verbal participation during music therapy sessions and engage in more social activities (Olderog-Millard & Smith, 1989). Other communication skills that show improvement over time when patients are engaged in a music therapy session include verbal feedback, smiling, eye contact, and meaningful participation (Pollack & Namazi, 1992). As individuals progress through the stages of Alzheimer's disease, music therapy interventions can be adapted to assist clients in maintaining their current level of functioning for as long as possible.

Caregivers can benefit from positive interactions fostered in music therapy sessions designed specifically for joint engagement between dementia patients and their loved ones. Dancing, rhythmic instrument playing, the singing of songs, movement to music, and instrumental ensembles are all examples of engaging activities that can bring together caregivers and patients. Caregivers who participated in music therapy sessions reported that they knew more positive ways to interact with their loved ones, felt more connected to their loved ones, recognized that music therapy activities were successful at achieving positive outcomes, and experienced satisfaction at the end of music therapy sessions (Clair & Ebberts, 1997; Clair, Tebb, & Bernstein, 1993; Hanser & Clair, 1995). Music is an intrinsic part of people's lives and therefore a familiar modality for fostering meaningful interactions between loved ones and their caregivers. Music can also provide opportunities for personal touch and positive physical interactions between individuals with dementia and others (Belgrave, 2009).

CONCLUSION

Music therapy has been recognized as one of the interventions most beneficial to individuals with Alzheimer's disease and other dementia-related disorders. Fortunately for such individuals, a musical background is not a prerequisite to the benefits music can provide. To address the progressive multi-faceted issues faced by patients, music therapists can design and implement music interventions to fit individuals' changing needs and functional abilities. Although a board-certified music therapist with specialized training in dementia-related disorders is preferred, there are important ways that other health-related professionals can employ music when a music therapist is not on duty or is otherwise unavailable. Positive outcomes are possible when using music interventions and will vary depending on the musical training of the provider. Care providers can successfully use music to induce sleep, prevent wandering, reduce agitation, relieve stress, manage pain, and improve mood. Professional music therapists are trained to address additional symptoms, such as the use of sensory stimulation to slow the decline of physical, psychological, and cognitive processes.

Carefully planned music therapy interventions can also do much to improve the quality of life for the families of loved ones affected by Alzheimer's disease and other dementia-related disorders. Family members often find that music provides a way of connecting to loved ones who are no longer able to use language for communication. Even without speech, singing appears to be relatively unaffected by the language processing difficulties associated with Alzheimer's disease. Families and caregivers can connect with their loved one by singing together an old familiar song. Having a moment of connection, even if a brief moment, is a gift for families who feel disconnected from their loved ones as they become more confused and disoriented. Singing, playing instruments, or dancing together prompt physical closeness between loved ones and allow for the sharing of emotions. Songs often cue memories of past holidays or family events that can be shared with loved ones. Such meaningful interactions can reduce the isolation felt by many individuals with Alzheimer's disease.

Music is a unique medium with the ability to engage multiple senses and areas of the brain simultaneously. It is capable of engaging people regardless of their cognitive abilities. Due to its familiarity and the fact that it is a medium enjoyed by nearly all individuals, music is generally quite successful in eliciting positive responses. With modern technology and the information provided in this text, healthcare providers will be able to address many of the needs experienced by their patients and loved ones experiencing the devastating effects of Alzheimer's disease. Music has become a valued component of care plans for individuals with all dementia-related disorders.

REFERENCES

Alzheimer's Association. (2010). Alzheimer's Association report: 2010 Alzheimer's disease facts and figures. *Alzheimer and Dementia, 6*, 158–194.

Alzheimer's Disease Education and Referral Center (ADEAR). (2008a). *Alzheimer's disease genetics fact sheet.* Retrieved from http://www.nia.nih.gov/Alzheimers/Publications/geneticsfs.htm

Alzheimer's Disease Education and Referral Center (ADEAR). (2008b). *The hallmarks of AD.* Retrieved from http://www.nia.nih.gov/Alzheimers/Publications/Unraveling/Part2/hallmarks.htm

Alzheimer's Disease Education and Referral Center (ADEAR). (2009). *Research findings benefit caregivers.* Retrieved from http://www.nia.nih.gov/Alzheimers/Publications/Unraveling/Part4/findings.htm

Alzheimer's Disease Education and Referral Center (ADEAR). (2010). *Alzheimer's disease fact sheet.* Retrieved from http://www.nia.nih.gov/Alzheimers/Publications/adfact.htm

Austrom, M. G., & Lu, Y. (2009). Long term caregiving: Helping families of persons with mild cognitive impairment cope. *Current Alzheimer's Research, 6*, 392–398.

Belgrave, M. (2009). The effect of expressive and instrumental touch on the behavior states of older adults with late-stage dementia of the Alzheimer's type and on music therapist's perceived rapport. *Journal of Music Therapy, 37,* 196–204.

Boyle, P. A., Buchman, A. S., Barnes, L. L., & Bennett, D. A. (2010). Effect of a purpose in life on risk of incident Alzheimer disease and mild cognitive impairment in community-dwelling older persons. *Archives of General Psychiatry, 67*(3), 304–310.

Brotons, M. (2003). Music therapy with Alzheimer's patients and their family caregivers: A pilot project. *Journal of Music Therapy, 40*, 138–150.

Brotons, M., & Pickett-Cooper, P. K. (1996). The effects of music therapy intervention on agitation behaviors of Alzheimer's disease patients. *Journal of Music Therapy, 33*(1), 2–18.

Carruth, E. K. (1997). The effects of singing and the spaced retrieval technique on improving face-name recognition in nursing home residents with memory loss. *Journal of Music Therapy, 34*(3), 165–186.

Cevasco, A. M., & Grant, R. E. (2003). Comparison of different methods for eliciting exercise-to-music for clients with Alzheimer's disease. *Journal of Music Therapy, 40*(1), 41–56.

Clair, A. A. (1996). The effect of singing on alert responses in persons with late stage dementia. *Journal of Music Therapy, 33*(4), 234–247.

Clair, A. A., & Bernstein, B. (1990). A comparison of singing, vibrotactile and nonvibrotactile instrumental playing responses in severely regressed persons with dementia of the Alzheimer's type. *Journal of Music Therapy, 27*(3), 119–125.

Clair, A. A., & Ebberts, A. G. (1997). The effects of music therapy on interactions between family caregivers and their care receivers with late stage dementia. *Journal of Music Therapy, 34*(3), 148–164.

Clair, A. A., Mathews, R. M., & Kosloski, K. (2005). Assessment of active music participation as an indication of subsequent music making engagement for persons with midstage dementia. *American Journal of Alzheimer's Disease and Other Dementias, 20*(1), 37–40.

Clair, A. A., Tebb, S., & Bernstein, B. (1993). The effects of socialization and music therapy intervention on self-esteem and loneliness in spouse caregivers of those diagnosed with dementia of the Alzheimer's type: A pilot study. *The American Journal of Alzheimer's Disease and Related Disorders and Research, 1,* 24–32.

Derwinger, A., Stigsdotter Neely, A., MacDonald, S., & Backman, L. (2005). Forgetting numbers in old age: Strategy and learning speed matter. *Gerontology, 51,* 277–284.

Dhooper, S. (1991). Caregivers of Alzheimer's disease patients: A review of the literature. *Journal of Gerontological Social Work, 18*, 19–37.

Gazzaley, A. (2009). *Normal aging.* Retrieved from http://memory.ucsf.edu/Education/Topics/normalaging.html

Gerdner, L. A. (1999). Individualized music intervention protocol. *Journal of Gerontological Nursing, 25*, 10–16.

Hampstead, B. M., Sathian, K., Moore, A. B., Nalisnick, C., & Stringer, A. Y. (2008). Explicit memory training leads to improved memory for face-name pairs in patients with mild cognitive impairment: Results of a pilot investigation. *Journal of the International Neuropsychological Society, 14*(5), 883–889.

Hanser, S., & Clair, A. A. (1995). Retrieving the losses of Alzheimer's disease for patients and caregivers with the aid of music. In T. Wigram, B. Saperston, & R. West (Eds.), *The art and science of music therapy: A handbook* (pp. 342–360). Switzerland: Harwood Academic.

Hanson, N., Gfeller, K., Woodworth, G., Swanson, E. A., & Garand, L. (1996). A comparison of the effectiveness of differing types and difficulty of music activities in programming for older adults with Alzheimer's disease and related disorders. *Journal of Music Therapy 33*(2), 93–123.

Jean, L., Bergeron, M. E., Thivierge, S., & Simard M. (2010). Cognitive intervention programs for individuals with mild cognitive impairment: Systematic review of the literature. *American Journal of Geriatric Psychiatry, 8*(4), 281–296.

Kaplan, M. (1996). *Clinical practice with caregivers of dementia patients.* Washington, DC: Taylor & Francis.

Kinsella, G. J., Mullaly, E., Rank, E., Ong, B., Burton, C., Price, S., Phillips, M., & Storey, E. (2009). Early intervention for mild cognitive impairment: A randomized controlled trial. *Journal of Neurology, Neurosurgery, and Psychiatry, 80*(7), 730–736.

Koger, S., Chapin, K., & Brotons, M. (1999). Is music therapy an effective intervention for dementia? A meta-analytic review of literature. *Journal of Music Therapy, 36*, 2–15.

Mariani, E., Monastero, R., & Mecocci, P. (2007). Mild cognitive impairment: A systematic review. *Journal of Alzheimers Disease, 12*(1), 23–35.

O'Connor, D. W., Ames, D., Gardner, B., & King, M. (2009). Psychosocial treatment of behavior symptoms in dementia: A systematic review of reports meeting quality standards. *International Psychogeriatrics, 21*(2), 225–240.

O'Hara, R., Brooks, J. O., III, Friedman, L., Schroder, C. M., Morgan, K. S., & Kraemer, H. C. (2007). Long-term effects of mnemonic training in community dwelling older adults. *Journal of Psychiatric Research, 41*, 585–590.

Olderog-Millard, K. A., & Smith, J. M. (1989). The influence of group singing therapy on the behavior of Alzheimer's disease patients. *Journal of Music Therapy, 26*(2), 58–70.

Pollack, N. J., & Namazi, K. H. (1992). The effect of music participation on the social behavior of Alzheimer's disease patients. *Journal of Music Therapy, 29*(1), 54–67.

Raglio, A., Bellelli, G., Traficante, D., Gianotti, M., Ubezio, M. C., Villani, D., et al. (2008). Efficacy of music therapy in the treatment of behavioral and psychiatric symptoms of dementia. *Alzheimer Disease & Associated Disorders, 22*, 158–162.

Smith, G. (1986). A comparison of the effects of three treatment interventions on cognitive functioning of Alzheimer patients. *Music Therapy, 6A*(1), 41–56.

Troyer, A. K., Murphy, K. J., Anderson, N. D., Moscovitch, M., & Craik, F. I. M. (2008). Changing everyday memory behavior in amnestic mild cognitive impairment: A randomized controlled trial. *Neuropsychological Rehabilitation 18*(1), 65–88.

Willis , S. L., Tennstedt, S. L., Marsiske, M., Ball, K., Elias, J., Koepke, K. M., Morris, J. N., Rebok, G. W., Unverzagt, F. W., Stoddard, A. M., & Wright, E. (2006). Long-term effects of cognitive training on everyday functional outcomes in older adults. *Journal of the American Medical Association, 296*, 2805–2814.

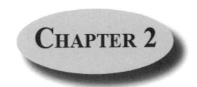

CHAPTER 2

REVIEW OF THE RESEARCH LITERATURE ON ALZHEIMER'S DISEASE AND MUSIC THERAPY

That song makes me want to jump up out of my seat! —Mr. B.

You could stay all day and sing and that would be fine by me. —Mrs. J.

INTRODUCTION

The uses of music to improve the lives of people who have Alzheimer's disease are vast and have been investigated for decades. The research literature shows that music and music therapy interventions have been employed to maintain and improve cognitive skills, decrease disruptive behaviors, and improve social and emotional needs of individuals who have Alzheimer's disease, as well as decrease caregiver stress. More specifically, music therapy interventions have been implemented to improve recall, maintain language skills, decrease problem behaviors such as physical agitation and wandering, maintain and improve active engagement, decrease isolation, and improve the quality of the relationship between the caregiver and the individual who has Alzheimer's disease (Brotons, Koger, & Pickett-Cooper, 1997; Koger, Chapin, & Brotons, 1999). This chapter provides a review of literature pertaining to the therapeutic outcomes obtained during music therapy sessions conducted with individuals who have Alzheimer's disease. The information synthesized in this chapter provides the rationale for the recommended music interventions outlined in the next chapter.

MUSIC THERAPY AND COGNITIVE SKILLS

As individuals progress through the stages of Alzheimer's disease, a decline in cognitive functioning occurs. Declines in memory, speech, orientation, attention, and an individual's level of engagement with the environment are gravely affected throughout the progression of Alzheimer's disease. Due to the degenerative nature of the disease, declines in cognitive skills will occur for all individuals who have Alzheimer's disease. Therefore, it is important to use various therapeutic techniques to maintain cognitive functioning for as long as possible. Music therapy interventions such as music-cued reminiscing, therapeutic singing, and musical mnemonic devices are often employed to maintain cognitive skills by using music to structure the environment and as a cue to recall information (Brotons et al., 1997; Koger et al., 1999).

A music-cued reminiscence intervention uses music as a structure and a cue to assist individuals in recalling and processing important events from their lives. Therapeutic singing uses familiar music to structure the environment and music therapy session. Therapeutic singing of familiar music can also be used to enhance an individual's orientation to reality. Hearing familiar music can increase an individual's ability to engage in the present moment and participate meaningfully with others. Therapeutic singing is also used to maintain an individual's functional language skills. Singing requires one to use the unique combination of language and melody. In addition, songs are stored in an area of the brain that is still accessible for individuals who can sing but might not otherwise speak. A musical mnemonic device pairs familiar music with new information to facilitate learning new material. For example, the melody of a familiar song such as "Bicycle Built for Two" can be paired with new information, such as a room number, to aid in recall of the new material. The lyrics of the first line, "Daisy, Daisy, give me your answer do," could be changed to "My room, my room, is 326" (Brotons et al., 1997; Carruth, 1997; Koger et al., 1999).

Bruer, Spitznagel, and Cloninger (2007) examined the effect of participation in a music therapy session on overall cognitive functioning for individuals diagnosed with dementia. Older adults participated in both the experimental condition of music therapy and the control condition. During the music therapy sessions, participants engaged in singing and instrument playing interventions, whereas during the control conditions participants watched familiar movies. In this study, participants' cognitive functioning was determined by the Mini-Mental State Exam (MMSE; Folstein, Folstein, & McHugh, 1975). The MMSE is a 30-question assessment that measures an individual's overall cognitive functioning, including orientation to time and place, attention, recall, and language. A high score of 25–30 indicates no cognitive decline. A score of 21–24 indicates that an individual has mild cognitive decline. A score of 10–20 indicates a moderate cognitive decline, and a score below 9 indicates severe cognitive decline. Cognitive functioning was measured prior to the experimental or control condition, upon completion of the experimental or control condition, and the following morning. Resulting MMSE scores showed improvements in participants' overall cognitive functioning by 2 points immediately after the music intervention and 3.69 points when measured the next morning; both increases in scores were significantly greater when compared with the MMSE scores of individuals after the movie-watching condition.

Similar results were found in an earlier study conducted by Smith (1986). The researcher sought to study the effect of three different interventions on three areas of cognitive functioning—orientation, attention, and language—as measured by the MMSE (Folstein et al., 1975). Participants received three conditions: (1) music-cued reminiscing sessions, (2) reminiscing sessions without music, and (3) music therapy sessions that did not use reminiscing interventions. Results showed that overall cognition scores improved for the third condition, music therapy sessions without reminiscing. Additionally, language scores improved for participants after the music-cued reminiscing sessions and the reminiscing sessions without music.

Brotons and Koger (2000) examined the effect of music-cued reminiscing sessions on speech content and fluency. Participants experienced the experimental condition—singing and music-cued reminiscing, and the control condition—reminiscing without music. Speech content and fluency were measured through the Western Aphasia Battery (WAB; Kertesz, 1982), which is used to assess language skills for individuals who have dementia. The WAB was completed by participants before the intervention, once after the music therapy intervention (experimental condition), and once after the control condition. Results showed a greater increase in participants' speech content and fluency after music-cued reminiscing sessions than after reminiscing sessions without music.

Another area of cognitive functioning affected by Alzheimer's disease is recall of newly learned information. The task of teaching an individual who has Alzheimer's disease new information is difficult; therefore, pairing new information in a familiar musical context can result in greater recall accuracy for the new information (Carruth, 1997; Prickett & Moore, 1991). Incorporating important information that a person needs to learn into a song may result in higher success for recalling the information than teaching new information in spoken formats. As individuals progress through the stages of Alzheimer's disease, they may have an increase in the number of caregivers that assist them with activities of daily living. Individuals who have Alzheimer's disease often have difficulty with face-name recognition, which can result in confusing the names of facility caregivers with family members or others (Reisberg & Franssen, 1999). An effective intervention for maintaining face-name recall in individuals who have Alzheimer's disease is the spaced retrieval technique. This technique uses shaping to learn and retain information in long-term memory (Abrahams & Camp, 1993; Camp, 1998). In this technique, an individual is presented an object and told the name of that specific item. The individual is then asked to recall the item when it is presented. The space between presentation and recall of the item is gradually increased, with an expectation that the information will be stored in long-term memory and can be recalled days or weeks later (Abrahams & Camp, 1993; Camp, 1998). Carruth (1997) examined the use of this memory-training technique paired with singing to increase face-name recognition in older adults with memory loss. The sample was comprised of older adults diagnosed with Alzheimer's disease, stroke, or chronic obstructive pulmonary disease. The participants were presented with pictures of staff members at their long-term care facility. The space between the picture presentation and recall was filled with singing. Each music condition was the same and consisted of singing twice a familiar song with new words. Results showed that three of four participants with Alzheimer's disease demonstrated improvement in face-name recall after music therapy sessions paired with the spaced retrieval technique.

The above-mentioned studies demonstrate the use of therapeutic singing, music-cued reminiscing, and music-mnemonic devices to aid in maintaining cognitive skills for individuals who have Alzheimer's disease. A more recent study showed that participation in exercise routines may also assist in maintaining cognitive functioning (Van de Winckel, Feys, De Weerdt, & Dom, 2004). Participants diagnosed with moderate to severe dementia were assigned to either an experimental condition of music-assisted exercise, or a control condition of daily conversations. Cognitive scores measured by the MMSE (Folstein et al., 1975) improved significantly for participants in the exercise condition. Participants who received the daily conversation sessions showed no significant improvements in MMSE scores.

MUSIC THERAPY AND ACTIVE ENGAGEMENT

Individuals often experience declines in levels of engagement with their environment as they progress through the stages of Alzheimer's disease. Therefore, an underlying therapeutic outcome of many music therapy interventions is to increase an individual's level of attention and participation. Common music therapy interventions employed with clients diagnosed with Alzheimer's disease include singing, moving to music, instrument playing, songwriting, and music-cued reminiscing (Brotons et al., 1997). Individuals in different stages respond to music therapy interventions differently; therefore, music therapists often use adaptations and variations of interventions and therapeutic outcomes to maximize client engagement. For example, an individual in the early stages of Alzheimer's disease can actively engage in singing interventions. However, as cognitive functioning declines, changes in active participation during singing interventions may occur. Music therapists can structure singing interventions to provide success for all clients, regardless of the progression of the illness. Instead of expecting the client to actively sing an entire verse of a familiar song, the music therapist may structure the song so that the participant has to fill in only one phrase or a single word to the familiar song.

Many factors such as instrument placement, intervention type, accompaniment instrument and pattern, and the use of live or recorded music can impact the engagement level of a client during a music therapy session. Music therapists often use instrument placement to foster the highest level of active participation for individuals. For example, clients may want to hold a drum in their hand and strike it with a mallet; however, if a vibrotactile instrument such as a drum with a responsive drum head is placed in a client's lap, they can feel the vibrations and are more likely to exhibit higher participatory responses (Clair & Bernstein, 1990).

Secondly, the type of music therapy intervention employed can also affect an individual's level of engagement during a music therapy session. Brotons and Pickett-Cooper (1994) examined the effect of five music therapy interventions—singing, instrument playing, moving to music, music games, and composing and improvising—on participation levels of individuals who had Alzheimer's disease. Participants reported that they enjoyed all interventions equally; however, they were more engaged during instrument playing and dancing interventions than composing and improvising. Hanson, Gfeller, Woodworth, Swanson, and Garand (1996) also examined participation levels during music therapy interventions. The researchers focused on individuals in the early and middle stages of Alzheimer's disease and employed three different music therapy interventions—singing, moving to music, and instrument playing—to determine their effectiveness for eliciting participation. Results showed that participants were more engaged during movement interventions and least engaged during singing interventions.

A more recent study conducted by Cevasco and Grant (2006) with individuals in the middle or late stage of dementia resulted in similar findings. Participants were more engaged during instrument playing and moving to music interventions than singing interventions. A secondary purpose of the study was to determine if there was a difference in the participation elicited by varying accompaniment instruments: djembe, acoustic guitar, autoharp, keyboard, unaccompanied singing, and guitar and djembe combined. The highest level of participation occurred during unaccompanied singing and djembe accompaniment conditions. The lowest level of participation occurred during guitar and djembe accompaniment together. The researchers suggested that the use of two accompaniment instruments together may have provided too much auditory stimulation for participants.

Other researchers have examined the frequency of alert responses during unaccompanied singing for individuals with late-stage dementia (Belgrave, 2009; Clair, 1996). Individuals who have late-stage dementia with no discernable language can still present discernable, purposeful responses to auditory stimulation. Clair (1996) examined the frequency of alert responses during three conditions: unaccompanied singing, newspaper reading, and silence. Alert responses were defined as vocalizations, opening of eyes, turning of one's head to localize sounds, and whole body movements. Alert responses occurred most frequently when participants listened to unaccompanied singing, followed by reading, with the fewest responses occurring while sitting silently. Belgrave (2009) found that pairing unaccompanied singing with a gentle touch to the arm, shoulder, or hand can increase alert behavior states as well, especially during the initial encounter an individual has with a music therapist.

Lastly, the accompaniment pattern and the use of live music can also affect individuals' level of participation in music therapy sessions. Groene (2001) examined the differences between live and recorded music and a simple or complex guitar accompaniment style on engagement levels of individuals in the middle and late stages of dementia. Results showed that live music with complex rhythms maintained the attention of individuals who had dementia at much higher rates than live music with simple rhythms, or recorded music with complex or simple rhythms. The use of live music is further supported by results of a study conducted by Holmes, Knights, Dean, Hodkinson, and Hopkins (2006). The researchers explored the effectiveness of live music on increasing engagement levels with individuals who had moderate to severe dementia. Each subject was randomly assigned to one of three conditions: live interactive music, pre-recorded music listening, or silent periods. Only 12.5% of subjects displayed positive engagement during the silent period. In the pre-recorded music sessions, only 25% showed positive engagement, which was not a significant increase from the silent period. However, 69% of subjects displayed a significant increase in positive engagement during live interactive music sessions, regardless of dementia severity. The findings emphasize the immediate effect live music can have on patients who have Alzheimer's disease at even the most severe level of cognitive impairment.

The evidence supporting live music does not preclude the use of recorded music with individuals who have Alzheimer's disease. Nursing home residents with Alzheimer's disease reported that they perceived increases in their level of alertness and happiness and they recalled past events more accurately after "Big Band" music was played during their recreational periods for 6 months, as compared to residents with similar diagnoses who participated in recreation groups working puzzles, drawing, and painting for the same 6 months (Lord & Garner, 1993). While some individuals who have Alzheimer's disease attentively participate in music activities, research indicates that they can increase their successful attentiveness with minimal guidance. Simply playing background music may increase pleasure or distract clients exhibiting negative behaviors, while other clients may benefit from structure and training provided by music therapists or other caregivers (Gregory, 2002).

MOVEMENT TO MUSIC

As the illness progresses, physical issues worsen for patients who have Alzheimer's disease. For individuals who have difficulty maintaining attention and alertness, increasing involvement in physical exercise becomes imperative to maintain their strength and flexibility. Increased movement and physical activity can help delay the rigidity and contractures of extremities and joints that set in toward the end stages of the disease (Reisberg & Franssen, 1999). Adding music to an exercise program can assist with maintaining attention and the compliance of participants. Several music interventions have shown positive results in eliciting high levels of participation during exercises (Cevasco & Grant, 2003; Groene, Zapchenk, Marble, & Kantar, 1998; Mathews, Clair, & Kosloski, 2001).

Recorded instrumental music designed to coordinate with set exercise routines can yield high participation rates from individuals who have Alzheimer's disease (Cevasco & Grant, 2003; Mathews et al., 2001). Cueing systems can also increase participation levels for exercise-to-music sessions with individuals who are in the early and middle stages of dementia. Cevasco and Grant (2003) found that continuous verbal cueing paired with easy movement tasks resulted in high levels of participation. Increased participation was also found when instrumental music was used, as opposed to music with singing. These studies illustrate different factors that can affect an individual's participation in a music therapy session.

ASSESSMENT OF ENGAGEMENT BEHAVIORS

Clair, Mathews, and Kosloski (2005b) found that the initial assessment of participation levels during various interventions can be an indicator of future levels of participation in sessions. The researchers observed participants in the middle stages of dementia during assessment sessions consisting of singing, physical exercise, and instrument playing. Participants were then labeled as immediate participators, ready participators, reluctant participators, or non-participators. Labels were based on their level of participation, which was defined as how many verbal prompts were needed to initiate participation. The findings showed that the initial assessment of participation was an accurate representation of participation across sessions of singing, physical exercise, and instrument playing. Performing initial assessments of participation level and knowing that those levels may remain constant across sessions can be useful for therapists when identifying therapeutic outcomes and implementation of music therapy interventions.

MUSIC THERAPY AND DISRUPTIVE BEHAVIORS

It is common for individuals who have Alzheimer's disease to display disruptive behaviors. These individuals' inability to express their feelings and confusion about tasks they are requested to perform can result in outbursts and other disruptive behaviors as they become agitated (Reisberg & Franssen, 1999). Disruptive behaviors can be demonstrated through using abusive language, throwing objects, kicking, and yelling. The research literature on the topic of agitation for patients who have Alzheimer's disease suggests that using an individual's preferred music instead of generally selected recorded music elicits the most calming behaviors (Casby & Holm, 1994; Heim, 2003; Sung & Chang, 2005; Sung, Chang, & Abbey, 2006). Having musical training earlier in life, such as playing in an ensemble or having private lessons, does not affect an individual's response to music interventions designed to decrease agitation. Regardless of musical training, individuals show reduced agitation during the music intervention as well as immediately after the sessions (Brotons & Pickett-Cooper, 1996). Reducing disruptive vocalizations can have a positive impact on the caregivers as well as increase the patient's quality of life and is therefore an area of much interest for researchers.

Bath times commonly are met with disruptive behaviors from an individual with dementia because of the resulting confusion when another person bathes that individual. Thomas, Heitman, and Alexander (1997) examined the effectiveness of recorded music during bath time to decrease disruptive behaviors for individuals diagnosed with Alzheimer's disease. Participant-preferred music was played during bathing periods, resulting in a decrease in agitation behaviors during that time. Researchers also noted that participants' quality of life increased and care providers' job satisfaction improved with the addition of music during bath times.

Clark, Lipe, and Bilbrey (1998) examined the use of preferred recorded music on aggressive behaviors during bath time. The researchers identified 15 possible aggressive behaviors to observe: yelling, abusive language, hitting, verbal resistance, crying, physical resistance, grabbing, pinching, kicking, spitting, wandering, biting, throwing, scratching, and gouging. Results showed that using preferred recorded music during bath time decreased the frequency of aggressive behaviors, elevated participants' mood, and increased participant cooperation.

Individuals who have Alzheimer's disease also display disruptive behaviors during mealtimes. Denney (1997) examined the effectiveness of background recorded music in decreasing disruptive behaviors during mealtimes. Results revealed that disruptive behaviors decreased when music was present. When music was withdrawn, participants' disruptive behaviors increased; when music was reintroduced, participants' disruptive behaviors decreased again. Goddaer and Abraham (1994) found similar results of declines in disruptive behaviors during mealtimes when background music was present. Outside of mealtime activity, using only relaxing or stimulative recorded music does not generally produce favorable results. Clair and Bernstein (1994) found that one of three listening conditions—stimulative music, sedative music, and no music—did not influence the frequency of agitated behaviors displayed by individuals who had severe dementia. When individuals who have Alzheimer's disease listen to their preferred music, they may experience a significant reduction in agitation levels as compared to times when they listen to classical music, listen to readings, or do not have a music intervention (Garland, Beer, Eppingstall, & O'Connor, 2007; Gerdner, 2000; Hicks-Moore & Robinson, 2008). Therefore, playing one type of music for all patients may not offer the personalization that elicits positive changes in agitation.

Disruptive behaviors also are demonstrated through wandering. Physical wandering from residences and within facilities is a dangerous occurrence that worsens as the disease progresses. Participation in music therapy sessions can decrease the amount of time spent wandering for individuals who have Alzheimer's disease. Groene (1993) compared the frequency of wandering behaviors during music therapy and reading sessions. Results revealed a larger decrease in the amount of wandering during music interventions than reading sessions, suggesting that music might hold an individual's attention for longer periods of time than reading.

MUSIC AND EMOTIONS

Individuals who have impaired cognition commonly experience frustration, apathy, lack of engagement with others, emotional outbursts, strained relationships with caregivers, depression, and decreased communication, which can result in a greatly decreased quality of life. Music therapy interventions can be used to increase mood as a result of the emotional connection inherent in music. Music can also provide structure and support for socialization to occur in a natural environment. Many individuals who have Alzheimer's disease feel isolated over time when they are unable to communicate effectively or understand what is happening around them. These feelings of isolation can lead to symptoms of depression and apathy. Depressive symptoms of individuals who have Alzheimer's disease, living in a residential care facility, can be reduced over time through participation in reminiscence-based music therapy groups (Ashida, 2000).

Both interactive music therapy sessions and passive music listening supervised by nurses have elicited positive social responses for individuals who have Alzheimer's disease. The types of social behaviors measured vary across studies but consistently show improvement. Increasing socialization among individuals who have Alzheimer's disease is one method to decrease feelings of isolation and apathy that are commonly seen with this population. Individuals who had middle-stage dementia engaged in more interactions with others during therapeutic singing groups than with reminiscing groups (Olderog-Millard & Smith, 1989). Additionally, active participation along with higher verbal and vocal participation during group times was found when individuals attended groups incorporating therapeutic singing.

Similar responses are seen for individuals who have early- and middle-stage dementia engaged in individual sessions that incorporate singing, movement, or instrument playing. Pollack and Namazi (1992) found that direct and indirect interactions with others increased during and after music therapy sessions. Specifically, individuals demonstrated an increase in smiling, eye contact, verbalizations, and participation. Also, caregivers perceived an improvement in their loved one's social and emotional areas after participating in music therapy sessions (Brotons & Marti, 2003).

Ziv, Granot, Hai, Dassa, and Haimov (2007) examined the use of background music on social and verbal behaviors of individuals who had Alzheimer's disease. Participants were observed during free time with and without the presence of familiar background music. Results revealed that individuals talked more after the passive music listening than during free time without background music. Differences were also found among participants in the amount of time spent socializing with other group members. Individuals listening to music engaged in appropriate socialization behaviors at higher rates. This study is encouraging for several reasons. Passive music listening is a very easy activity to implement and requires no musical training. Very little cost and time are needed to conduct such an activity group. Finally, the outcomes of increased verbalizations and appropriate socialization behaviors are important client goals. While music familiar to individuals can be used as general background music to increase positive social behaviors and decrease negative behaviors related to agitation, many more targeted interventions have been investigated and indicate benefits for the individuals who have Alzheimer's disease and their caregivers.

CAREGIVER INTERACTIONS

Families and facility staff members who provide care for individuals who have Alzheimer's disease are faced with challenges as they respond to the physical, emotional, social, and cognitive needs of the individual. The high demands placed on caregivers can result in fatigue, exhaustion, depression, isolation, financial stress, and family pressures (Austrom & Lu, 2009; Dhooper, 1991; Kaplan, 1996). The need for alternative methods for engaging patients, staff, and families in positive interactions has resulted in an increase in the number of research studies investigating this topic. Music is a low-cost and accessible modality that can foster interactions for patient, families, and staff. General music and music therapy interventions can have positive effects on individuals who have Alzheimer's disease and their caregivers, which include

1. an increase in caregivers' self-esteem (Clair & Bernstein, 1993; Clair & Ebberts, 1997);

2. an increase in caregivers' satisfaction with time spent with their loved ones and their perceived amount of time spent in purposeful interactions with each other (Clair & Bernstein, 1993; Clair & Ebberts, 1997);

3. an increase in the number of touches caregivers initiate with their loved ones who, in return, are more responsive to the touch (Clair, 2002b; Clair & Ebberts, 1997);

4. a decrease in agitated daytime and nighttime behaviors (Clair, 2002a; Gerdner, 2005; Brown, Götell, & Ekman, 2001);

5. an increase in engagement in purposeful activities (Clair & Ebberts, 1997; Götell, Brown, & Ekman, 2003; Mathews & Kosloski, 2000).

USING MUSIC IN THE HOME

Individuals who have late-stage dementia and their caregivers can experience increased interactions when caregivers are trained to use music in the home. The frequency of positive interactions increases when music is chosen based on the preferred music of the individual who has Alzheimer's disease. Caregivers who have been trained by music therapists to use music in the home with their loved ones reported feeling comfortable using music activities and indicated that they planned to continue using music upon completion of the training (Clair, 2002b). Music therapy sessions that foster interactions between individuals who have Alzheimer's disease and their spouse and/or caregivers can have a positive impact on self-esteem, the satisfaction with time spent with loved ones, and the perceived amounts of time spent in purposeful interactions with each other. Music therapy activities, such as group singing, can help individuals who have Alzheimer's disease to engage with their spouses. Instrument playing has resulted in the highest level of engagement with spouses for individuals who have late-stage dementia (Clair & Bernstein, 1993; Clair & Ebberts, 1997).

When interacting with loved ones who have Alzheimer's disease, caregivers may experience aggressive and disruptive behaviors, resulting in a decline in touch and physical proximity. Participating in music therapy sessions can help caregivers initiate touch more frequently with their loved ones, who, in return, are more responsive to the touch (Clair & Ebberts, 1997). Another meaningful interaction that results in increased physical proximity for spouses caring for late-stage dementia patients is dancing to music. Dancing can provide a positive means of close physical contact when other types of contact are uncomfortable. When an individual loses the strength to stand, dancing can be modified by engaging in seated dances. Interlocking arms and swaying to music, using cheek-to-cheek proximity, and hugging from behind the seated person are modified options for dancing and maintaining positive physical touch between couples (Clair, 2002a). Even staff with no musical training can easily use the patient's preferred dance music.

STAFF USE OF MUSIC WITHIN FACILITIES

After participation in five training sessions, caregiver staff was able to successfully lead music sessions with individuals who had middle-stage dementia. Training sessions included music applications, how to lead a session, data collection methods, feedback, and recommendations for improvement. Caregiver staff was also able to determine engagement levels in the sessions for all participants. Levels of engagement for individuals who had middle-stage dementia during rhythm activities, movement activities, and singing activities were similar, whether led by a music therapist or by the facility activity staff with little to no formal music training (Clair, Mathews, & Kosloski, 2005a).

Clair (2002c) described an additional music-based protocol that can be easily administered by caregivers with no musical abilities to manage agitated behaviors shown by individuals who have late-stage dementia. When patients exhibit a cycle of agitation that occurs at a pinpointed time of day or night, the cycle can be interrupted by creating a "musical timeout." Dimming the lights, playing sedative, patient-preferred music for at least 30 minutes, and modeling sitting in a chair while encouraging the patient to do the same can increase physical relaxation to prevent the disruptive behavior from occurring. Beginning 30 to 40 minutes before a pinpointed agitation time and singing familiar songs with a patient for 15 to 20 minutes can also provide an interruption for the outbursts. Progressive muscle relaxation paired with sedative preferred music works well to physically relax a patient before a pinpointed aggressive behavior occurs. After turning on the sedative music, caregivers can verbally instruct the patient to tense each muscle or group of muscles for a period of 4 to 5 seconds and then release and relax the muscles for a period of 4 to 5 seconds. Many times, caregivers providing a model for muscle tension and release will aid the patient in engaging appropriately in progressive muscle relaxation.

Caregiver staff can also successfully implement rhythmic music interactions with individuals who have Alzheimer's disease after attending brief trainings led by music therapists. Mathews and Kosloski (2000) observed engagement levels of individuals who had Alzheimer's disease during rhythmic music therapy activities. Caregiver staff who attended a brief training on how to lead rhythmic music interventions then were observed while leading individual and group sessions. Patients' rate of engagement increased after the staff members attended the training, regardless of the level of dementia for each patient. Training sessions are a low-cost way to provide a positive option for caregiver staff to interact with patients.

When surveyed, nursing home staff reported using music successfully to calm agitated patients who have Alzheimer's disease, but they preferred to choose the specific music. Radios and televisions played as background noise are perceived by staff to trigger stress for patients as well as staff members (Ragneskog & Kihlgren, 1997). While performing their daily care routines, staff members can have positive impacts when they incorporate background music or sing to their patients who have Alzheimer's disease. Patients respond more often to singing than to background music, but both uses of music aid patients in displaying straightened posture, stronger and more symmetric movements, and a greater awareness of themselves and their environment. Patients are also able to perform tasks of daily living with intention, purpose, and competence that they had seemingly lost before the initiation of background music or singing from the staff (Götell et al., 2003). When staff engages in Music-Therapeutic Caregiving (MTC) through singing to the patient, the patient's compliance, cognition, and emotional areas can be improved, the quality of patient care can increase, and the caregiver–patient relationship can improve (Brown et al., 2001).

STAFF AND FAMILY JOINT USES OF MUSIC

In residential care facilities, Alzheimer's patients' levels of agitation and socialization can be positively affected when both staff and family members use music. Staff and family members can be trained on the appropriate uses of music to reduce agitation. Staff members can target the 30-minute window before individuals typically have their peak agitation periods to play music. Family members can play music during their visits to increase positive interactions and associations with music. Gerdner (2005) found that upon completion of training, staff and family members were successful in using music protocols to decrease agitation behaviors displayed by individuals who had Alzheimer's disease.

LONG-TERM EFFECTS OF MUSIC THERAPY

Studies conducted with individuals who have Alzheimer's disease commonly explore short-term responses and behavioral benefits received from music interventions. However, researchers are beginning to explore the long-term physiological benefits from weekly music therapy interventions. Takahashi and Matsushita (2006) examined the effect of weekly music therapy on systolic blood pressure and intelligence assessments. During a 2-year period, individuals who had moderate to severe dementia participated in weekly music therapy sessions and were compared with individuals who had similar levels of decline but did not participate in music therapy sessions. Results revealed that participants in the music therapy group had significantly lower systolic blood pressure and better intelligence scores than individuals in the non-music group. These results are encouraging, because systolic blood pressure typically increases with age and cognitive function declines with age for individuals who have dementia.

Kumar et al. (1999) examined the effect of participation in music therapy sessions over 4 months on relaxation as evidenced by the presence of neurotransmitters and neurohormones. Melatonin, norepinephrine, epinephrine, serotonin, and prolactin were measured after music therapy sessions. The researchers found an increase in melatonin levels for individuals who had Alzheimer's disease when compared to those who participated in the non-music group. Melatonin was found to increase further until 6 weeks post music therapy sessions. Researchers concluded that increased melatonin levels may have contributed to the relaxed and calm moods displayed by the participants. Similarly, a researcher examined the long-term benefits of participating in music therapy on disruptive behaviors in individuals who had Alzheimer's disease. Results revealed that a decline in disruptive behaviors was maintained for 1 month after participation in music therapy sessions for these individuals (Raglio et al., 2008). As more studies explore the long-term effects of music therapy and the ability to maintain gains over time, a clearer picture will begin to emerge about the most appropriate intervention techniques to use for optimal benefits.

CONCLUSION

Music interventions have far-reaching, positive impacts for individuals who have Alzheimer's disease, their families, and the staff who provide care. Music interventions can be used to decrease agitation, decrease disruptive behaviors, engage in reminiscence with others, improve functional language, increase mood, increase socialization, aid in reality orientation, and improve caregiver interactions. The many challenges faced by patients, families, and staff have resulted in the development of several music-based protocols. These protocols have been examined by researchers to determine the effectiveness in using music-based interventions to assist with challenges related to caring for an individual who has Alzheimer's disease. Unlike some intervention-based protocols in related fields that work for improving all patient speech patterns or mobility functions, music intervention protocols are most often individualized for each patient interaction. The literature pertaining to music and Alzheimer's disease supports the use of each patient's preferred music during interventions to optimize the individual's therapeutic outcome for most goal areas. This can present challenges to staff members who are not familiar with a wide variety of songs or music genres. The literature discussed in this chapter also supports the technique of training staff members who have little to no previous formal music training to implement music therapy interventions with success.

For this reason, the following chapter provides intervention activities, targeting a wide variety of goals, for families, staff, and music therapists to use with patients who have Alzheimer's disease. By incorporating music into more care routines for people with impaired cognition, the overall quality of life for patients, staff, and family members can increase. The result of improving patient care, improving family and spousal relationships, and optimizing behavioral, physical, emotional, and cognitive outcomes through music can transform current healthcare practices. Making music a part of patient healthcare is a low-cost, accessible intervention tool available for anyone who has the desire for change.

REFERENCES

Abrahams, J. P., & Camp, J. A. (1993). Maintenance and generalization of object naming training in anomia associated with degenerative dementia. *Clinical Gerontologist, 12*(3), 57–72.

Ashida, S. (2000). The effect of reminiscence music therapy sessions on changes in depressive symptoms in elderly persons with dementia. *Journal of Music Therapy, 37*, 170–182.

Austrom, M. G., & Lu, Y. (2009). Long term caregiving: Helping families of persons with mild cognitive impairment cope. *Current Alzheimer Research, 6*, 392–398.

Belgrave, M. (2009). The effect of expressive and instrumental touch on the behavior states of older adults with late-stage dementia of the Alzheimer's type and on music therapist's perceived rapport. *Journal of Music Therapy, 46*, 132–146.

Brotons, M., & Koger, S. M. (2000). The impact of music therapy on language functioning in dementia. *Journal of Music Therapy, 37*(3), 183–195.

Brotons, M., Koger, S. M., & Pickett-Cooper, P. (1997). Music and dementias: A review of literature. *Journal of Music Therapy, 34*, 204–245.

Brotons, M., & Marti, P. (2003). Music therapy with Alzheimer's patients and their family caregivers: A pilot project. *Journal of Music Therapy, 40*, 138–150.

Brotons, M., & Pickett-Cooper, P. (1994). Preferences of Alzheimer's disease patients for music activities singing, instruments, dance/movement, games, and composition/improvisation. *Journal of Music Therapy, 31*, 220–233.

Brotons, M., & Pickett-Cooper, P. K. (1996). The effects of music therapy intervention on agitation behaviors of Alzheimer's disease patients. *Journal of Music Therapy, 33*(1), 2–18.

Brown, S., Götell, E., & Ekman, S. L. (2001). "Music-therapeutic caregiving": The necessity of active music-making in clinical care. *The Arts in Psychotherapy, 28*(2), 125–135.

Bruer, R. A., Spitznagel, E., & Cloninger, C. R. (2007). The temporal limits of cognitive change from music therapy in elderly persons with dementia or dementia-like cognitive impairment: A randomized controlled trial. *Journal of Music Therapy, 44*, 308–328.

Camp, C. J. (1998). Facilitation of new learning in Alzheimer's disease. In G. C. Gilmore, P. J. Whitehouse, & M. L. Wykle (Eds.), *Memory, aging, and dementia, theory, assessment, and treatment* (pp. 212–225). New York: Springer.

Carruth, E. K. (1997). The effects of singing and the spaced retrieval technique on improving face-name recognition in nursing home residents with memory loss. *Journal of Music Therapy, 34*(3), 165–186

Casby, J. A., & Holm, M. B. (1994). The effect of music on repetitive disruptive vocalizations of persons with dementia. *The American Journal of Occupational Therapy, 48*, 883–889.

Cevasco, A. M., & Grant, R. E. (2003). Comparison of different methods for eliciting exercise-to-music for clients with Alzheimer's disease. *Journal of Music Therapy, 40*(1), 41–56.

Cevasco, A. M., & Grant, R. E. (2006). Value of musical instruments used by the therapist to elicit responses from individuals in various stages of Alzheimer's disease. *Journal of Music Therapy, 43*, 226–246.

Clair, A. A. (1996). The effect of singing on alert responses in persons with late-stage dementia. *Journal of Music Therapy, 33*(4), 234–247.

Clair, A. A. (2002a). Dance for emotional intimacy: Simple one-to-one interventions for family caregivers with loved ones in late-state dementia. *Activities Directors' Quarterly for Alzheimer's and Other Dementia Patients, 3*(3), 33–41.

Clair, A. A. (2002b). The effects of music therapy on engagement in family caregiver and care receiver couples with dementia. *American Journal of Alzheimer's Disease and Other Dementias, 17*(5), 286–290.

Clair, A. A. (2002c). Practical ways to use music to manage agitated behaviors in late-stage dementia. *Activities Directors' Quarterly for Alzheimer's and Other Dementia Patients, 3*(1), 41–48.

Clair, A. A., & Bernstein, B. (1990). A comparison of singing, vibrotactile and nonvibrotactile instrumental playing responses in severely regressed persons with dementia of the Alzheimer's type. *Journal of Music Therapy, 27*(3), 119–125.

Clair, A. A., & Bernstein, B. (1993). Effects of a socialization and music therapy intervention on self-esteem and loneliness in spouse caregivers of those diagnosed with dementia of the Alzheimer type: A pilot study. *American Journal of Alzheimer's Care and Related Disorders and Research, 8*(1), 24–32.

Clair, A. A., & Bernstein, B. (1994). The effect of no music, stimulative background music and sedative background music on agitated behaviors in persons with severe dementia. *Activities, Adaptation & Aging, 19*(1), 61–70.

Clair, A. A., & Ebberts, A. G. (1997). The effects of music therapy on interactions between family caregivers and their care receivers with late stage dementia. *Journal of Music Therapy, 34*(3), 148–164.

Clair, A. A., Mathews, R. M., & Kosloski, K. (2005a). Assessing active music participation of persons with midstage dementia. *Activities Directors' Quarterly for Alzheimer's and Other Dementia Patients, 6*(2), 15–22.

Clair, A. A., Mathews, R. M., & Kosloski, K. (2005b). Assessment of active music participation as an indication of subsequent music making engagement for persons with midstage dementia. *American Journal of Alzheimer's Disease and Other Dementias, 20*(1), 37–40.

Clark, M. E., Lipe, A. W., & Bilbrey, M. (1998). Use of music to decrease aggressive behaviors in people with dementia. *Journal of Gerontological Nursing, 24*(7), 10–-17.

Denney, A. (1997). Quiet music: An intervention for mealtime agitation? *Journal of Gerontological Nursing, 2*(7), 16–23.

Dhooper, S. (1991). Caregivers of Alzheimer's disease patients: A review of the literature. *Journal of Gerontological Social Work, 18*, 19–37.

Folstein, M. F., Folstein, S. E., & McHugh, P. R. (1975). Mini-mental state: A practical method for grading the cognitive state of patients for the clinician. *Journal of Psychiatric Research, 12*, 189–198.

Garland, K., Beer, E., Eppingstall, B., & O'Connor, D. W. (2007). Comparison of two treatments of agitated behavior in nursing home residents with dementia: Simulated family presence and preferred music. *American Journal of Geriatric Psychiatry, 15*(6), 514–521.

Gerdner, L. A. (2000). Effects of individualized versus classical "relaxation" music on the frequency of agitation in elderly persons with Alzheimer's disease and related disorders. *International Psychogeriatrics, 12*(1), 49–65.

Gerdner, L. A. (2005). Use of individualized music by trained staff and family: Translating research into practice. *Journal of Gerontological Nursing, 31*(6), 22–30.

Goddaer, J., & Abraham, I. L. (1994). Effects of relaxing music on agitation during meals among nursing home residents with severe cognitive impairment. *Archives of Psychiatric Nursing, 8*(3), 150–158.

Götell, E., Brown, S., & Ekman, S. L. (2003). Influence of caregiver singing and background music on posture, movement, and sensory awareness in dementia care. *International Psychogeriatrics, 15*(4), 411–430.

Gregory, D. (2002). Music listening for maintaining attention of older adults with cognitive impairments. *Journal of Music Therapy, 39*, 244–264.

Groene, R. W. (1993). Effectiveness of music therapy 1:1 intervention with individuals having senile dementia of the Alzheimer's type. *Journal of Music Therapy, 30*, 138–157.

Groene, R. (2001). The effect of presentation and accompaniment styles on attentional and responsive behaviors of participants with dementia diagnoses. *Journal of Music Therapy, 38*, 36–50.

Groene, R., Zapchenk, S., Marble, G., & Kantar, S. (1998). The effect of therapist and activity characteristics on the purposeful responses of probable Alzheimer's disease participants. *Journal of Music Therapy, 35*, 119–136.

Hanson, N., Gfeller, K., Woodworth, G., Swanson, E. A., & Garand, L. (1996). A comparison of the effectiveness of differing types and difficulty of music activities in programming for older adults with Alzheimer's disease and related disorders. *Journal of Music Therapy 33*(2), 93–123.

Heim, C. (2003). Effects of ambient baroque music on patients with dementia. *Australasian Journal on Ageing, 22*(4), 211–212.

Hicks-Moore, S., & Robinson, B. (2008). Favorite music and hand massage: Two interventions to decrease agitation in residents with dementia. *Dementia, 7*(1), 95–108.

Holmes, C., Knights, A., Dean, C., Hodkinson, S., & Hopkins, V. (2006). Keep music live: Music and the alleviation of apathy in dementia subjects. *International Psychogeriatrics, 18*(4), 623–630.

Kaplan, M. (1996). *Clinical practice with caregivers of dementia patients.* Washington, DC: Taylor & Francis.

Kertesz, A. (1982). *Western Aphasia Battery.* New York: Grune and Stratton.

Koger, S. M., Chapin, K., & Brotons, M. (1999). Is music therapy an effective intervention for dementia? A meta-analytic review of literature. *Journal of Music Therapy, 36*, 2–15.

Kumar, A. M., Tims, F., Cruess, D. G., Mintzer, M. T., Ironson, G., Loewenstein, D., Cattan, R., Fernandez, J. B., Eisdorfer, C., & Kumar, M. (1999). Music therapy increases serum melatonin levels in patients with Alzheimer's disease. *Alternative Therapies in Health and Medicine, 6*, 49–57.

Lord, T. R., & Garner, J. E. (1993). Effects of music on Alzheimer patients. *Perceptual and Motor Skills, 76*(2), 451–455.

Mathews, R. M., Clair, A. A., & Kosloski, K. (2001). Keeping the beat: Use of rhythmic music during exercise activities for the elderly with dementia. *American Journal of Alzheimer's Disease and Other Dementias, 16*(6), 377–380.

Mathews, R. M., & Kosloski, R. K. (2000). Brief in-service training in music therapy for activity aides: Increasing engagement of persons with dementia in rhythm activities. *Activities, Adaptation and Aging, 24*(4), 41–49.

Olderog-Millard, K. A., & Smith, J. M. (1989). The influence of group singing therapy on the behavior of Alzheimer's disease patients. *Journal of Music Therapy, 26*(2), 58–70.

Pollack, N. J., & Namazi, K. H. (1992). The effect of music participation on the social behavior of Alzheimer's disease patients. *Journal of Music Therapy, 29*(1), 54–67.

Prickett, C. A., & Moore, R. S. (1991). The use of music to aid memory of Alzheimer's patients. *Journal of Music Therapy, 28*(2), 101–110.

Raglio, A., Bellelli, G., Traficante, D., Gianotti, M., Ubezio, M. C., Villani, D., & Trabucchi, M. (2008). Efficacy of music therapy in the treatment of behavioral and psychiatric symptoms of dementia. *Alzheimer Disease & Associated Disorders, 22*, 158–162.

Ragneskog, H., & Kihlgren, M. (1997). Music and other strategies to improve the care of agitated patients with dementia. *Scandinavian Journal of Caring Sciences, 11*, 176–182.

Reisberg, B., & Franssen, E. H. (1999). Clinical stages of Alzheimer's disease. In M. J. deLeon (Ed.), *An atlas of Alzheimer's disease* (pp. 11–20). New York: Parthenon.

Smith, G. (1986). A comparison of the effects of three treatment interventions on cognitive functioning of Alzheimer patients. *Music Therapy, 6A*(1), 41–56.

Sung, H. C., & Chang, A. M. (2005). Use of preferred music to decrease agitated behaviors in older people with dementia: A review of the literature. *Journal of Clinical Nursing, 14*(9), 1133–1140.

Sung, H. C., Chang, A. M., & Abbey, J. (2006). The effects of preferred music on agitation of older people with dementia in Taiwan. *International Journal of Geriatric Psychiatry, 21*(10), 999–1000.

Takahashi, T., & Matsushita, H. (2006). Long-term effects of music therapy on elderly with moderate/severe dementia. *Journal of Music Therapy, 43*, 317–333.

Thomas, D., Heitman, R., & Alexander, T. (1997). The effects of music on bathing cooperation for residents with dementia. *Journal of Music Therapy, 34*, 246–259.

Van de Winckel, A., Feys, H., De Weerdt, W., & Dom, R. (2004). Cognitive and behavioral effects of music-based exercises in patients with dementia. *Clinical Rehabilitation, 18*(3), 253–260.

Ziv, N., Granot, A., Hai, S., Dassa, A., & Haimov, I. (2007). The effect of background stimulative music on behavior in Alzheimer's patients. *Journal of Music Therapy, 44*, 329–343.

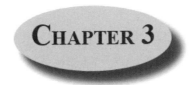

CHAPTER 3

CLINICAL APPLICATIONS FOR ALZHEIMER'S DISEASE AND RELATED DISORDERS

FOCUS AREA 1: ADDRESSING COGNITIVE NEEDS WITH MUSIC

The primary symptom of Alzheimer's disease is a decline in cognitive functioning. As the disease progresses, a person experiences changes in speech, memory, and ability to focus attention. The findings of numerous research studies indicate that music therapy interventions can assist in maintaining cognitive skills of individuals who have Alzheimer's disease (Brotons & Koger, 2000; Caruth, 1997; Prickett & Moore, 1991; Smith, 1986). The following learning activities use music to facilitate short-term and long-term memory recall, improve face-name recognition, and maintain focus of attention.

Clinical Application 1.1

Target Behavior: Long-term memory retrieval

Music: Chosen from a variety of genres and time periods; specifically, songs that were popular during the individual's teenage to young adult years.

Level 1—General Staff

Directions: Choose several different songs from CDs or MP3 files that contain lyrics describing popular events in history, that review an individual's life, or that were commonly played in social settings such as dances (see Reminiscence song recommendations). Play selected songs for the group, alternating genres and topics. After listening to a song, ask individuals what that song reminds them of or what things come to mind.

Level 2—Volunteer Musician

Directions: Divide the group of participants into two teams. Then provide the melody line of a song by humming or playing it on an instrument such as piano or guitar. The team that guesses the song title or can recite the largest portion of the text of the song correctly receives an "X" or an "O" for their team. Immediately after singing the entire song with live accompaniment, lead a reminiscence discussion about the time period brought to mind for each person. Ask questions such as, "Where were you when you heard that song?" "What were you doing when that song was played?" "Who do you remember singing that song?"

Level 3—Board-Certified Music Therapist

Activity Name: "Tic Tac Tune"

Other Goals Addressed: Cognitive Stimulation through Problem Solving, Improved Short-term Memory and Improved Sequencing, Increased Autonomy, Purposeful Participation, Socialization

Directions: Divide the group of participants into two teams. Then provide the melody line of a song by humming or playing it on an instrument such as piano or guitar. The team that guesses the song title or can recite the largest portion of the text of the song correctly receives an "X" or an "O" for their team. Immediately after singing the entire song with live accompaniment, lead a reminiscence discussion about the time period brought to mind for each person. Ask questions such as, "Where were you when you heard that song?" "What were you doing when that song was played?" "Who do you remember singing that song?" Assess the individuals who are having difficulty participating in the conversations (due to confusion) and modify the question/answer format to maximize each participant's interaction. Assess engagement of each participant as the group progresses and direct questions to and elicit responses from individuals who are having difficulty engaging at different points in the session. Monitor changes in participation levels for individuals from week to week to note decline, maintenance of, or improvement in skills.

Clinical Application 1.2

Target Behavior: Face-name recognition

Music: Chosen from a variety of genres and time periods; specifically, songs that were popular during the individual's teenage to young adult years. Selected songs should have notable themes that could represent people in the group (see Thematic song recommendations).

Level 1—General Staff

Directions: Choose several different songs from CDs or MP3 files that have thematic lyrics in categories such as dancing, feeling happy, cars, military service, etc. After each song is played, ask group members to point to and name someone in the group that song reminds them of.

Level 2—Volunteer Musician

Directions: Make a performance list from your repertoire that groups songs with thematic lyrics into categories such as dancing, feeling happy, cars, military service, etc. After each song is played, ask group members to point to and name someone in the group that song reminds them of.

Level 3—Board-Certified Music Therapist

Activity Name: "Face-Name Jeopardy"

Other Goals Addressed: Cognitive Stimulation through Problem Solving, Improved Short-term Memory and Improved Sequencing, Increased Autonomy, Purposeful Participation, Socialization

Directions: This activity is most successful if caregivers are involved in the process of creating the game board.* Interview caregivers in order to identify meaningful people in each client's life. Ask caregivers to bring in pictures of those people or take pictures of loved ones while they are visiting the client. If possible, find out if there are songs the loved ones can recall that remind them of the client. Create a game board using a large piece of foam board (can be scored for easy folding/storage). Create 4 to 5 columns labeled with various social groupings of people (Friends, Family, Staff, Neighbors, Me!) and 5 to 6 rows of cards with the names of songs for each row on one side and a picture of a client's loved one, staff, or self on the other side. Each client will take turns choosing (1) a social grouping, and (2) a song title. When the song title is chosen, turn the card over and show the group the picture of the individual on the back. Then take the picture to that client and ask him/her to identify the person in the picture (if this task is beyond the client's cognitive ability level, adapt the activity by stating the name of the person in the picture to the client and watch for signs of recognition). Then share with the group the name of the person in the picture, the significance of this person to the client, and why the song reminds this loved one of the client. If it is a staff member's photo, tell the group why that song is his/her favorite song and what it reminds the staff member of. Then ask if anyone can recall the melody line (verse or chorus) for the song and then sing the entire song as a group, encouraging participation and instrument play.

*Adaptation: If caregivers are not able to assist with this activity, modify the activity board to include pictures of only residents and staff members.

Clinical Application 1.3

Target Behavior: Improved problem solving

Music: Chosen from a variety of genres and time periods; specifically, songs that were popular during the individual's teenage to young adult years. Selected songs should have unique or easily recognized titles (see Thematic song recommendations).

Level 1—General Staff

Directions: Choose several different songs from CDs or MP3 files that have song titles that are recognizable and unique (e.g., "Crazy," "Swing Low, Sweet Chariot," "Fly Me to the Moon"). Before you play each song, ask group members to guess which song they are about to hear by giving them clues for each song title. Encourage participation from everyone in the group.

Level 2—Volunteer Musician

Directions: Make a performance list from your repertoire of songs that have unique and recognizable titles (e.g., "Crazy," "Swing Low, Sweet Chariot," "Fly Me to the Moon"). Before you play each song, ask group members to guess which song they are about to hear by giving them clues for each song title. Encourage participation from everyone attending the group music time.

Level 3—Board-Certified Music Therapist

Activity Name: "Musical Map Puzzle"

Other Goals Addressed: Improved Short-term Memory, Improved Sequencing, Increased Autonomy, Purposeful Participation, Socialization

Directions: Cut a wall-sized map of the United States into puzzle pieces that have songs corresponding with particular parts of the country (e.g., a Beach Boys song for California). The number of puzzle pieces can vary depending on the number of group participants, or the amount of time you have to lead the group. Each person is given one puzzle piece. The client must first decide where to fit the puzzle piece into the map. Next, give a song clue and the client must match the song clue with the regional clue on the back of the puzzle piece to guess the song. After the correct song is guessed (with help from other group members, if needed), sing the song while providing chordal accompaniment. Music therapy techniques such as chaining, modeling, and structuring can be used to elicit optimum involvement from all group members.

Clinical Application 1.4

Target Behavior: Long-term memory retrieval

Music: Chosen from a variety of genres and time periods; specifically, songs that were popular during the individual's teenage to young adult years. Selected songs should have notable melodic contours.

Level 1—General Staff

Directions: Choose several different songs from CDs or MP3 files that have catchy and recognizable openings/intros. Play the beginning of each song and encourage the group participants to work together to remember the name of the song or lyrics from the song. Successive approximations should be celebrated, such as remembering the words to the chorus.

Level 2—Volunteer Musician

Directions: Create a game board using a large piece of foam board cut in the shape of a pyramid. Label each section of the pyramid with a clue about each song category or genre such as "Songs about Water" or "Songs from the 40's." Attach a packet of song titles to each category/section of the pyramid using clear plastic binders cut to the desired size and stapled to the board. Take turns having each group participant draw a song card from the clue category of their choice. At this point, give the person another clue about the song and encourage the resident to pair the two clues together, using the similarities to identify the song title. After the song title is identified, sing the song while providing chordal accompaniment.

Level 3—Board-Certified Music Therapist

Activity Name: "Music Pyramid"

Other Goals Addressed: Cognitive Stimulation through Problem Solving, Improved Short-term Memory and Improved Sequencing, Increased Autonomy, Purposeful Participation, Socialization

Directions: Create a game board using a large piece of foam board cut in the shape of a pyramid. Label each section of the pyramid with a clue about each song category or genre such as "Songs about Water" or "Songs from the 40's." Attach a packet of song titles to each category/section of the pyramid using clear plastic binders cut to the desired size and stapled to the board. Take turns having each group participant draw a song card from the clue category of their choice. At this point, give the person another clue about the song and encourage the resident to pair the two clues together, using the similarities to identify the song title. After the song title is identified, sing the song while providing chordal accompaniment. Music therapy techniques such as chaining, modeling, and structuring can be used to elicit optimum involvement from all group members. Assess the individuals who are having difficulty participating in the conversations (due to confusion) and modify the question/answer format to maximize each participant's interaction. Assess each participant's level of engagement as the group progresses. Direct questions to and elicit responses from individuals who are having difficulty engaging at different points in the session. Monitor changes in participation levels for individuals from week to week to note decline, maintenance of, or improvement in skills.

FOCUS AREA 2: ADDRESSING DISRUPTIVE BEHAVIORS WITH MUSIC

The individual who has Alzheimer's disease often experiences behavior changes as the illness progresses. Aggressive behaviors such as yelling, abusive language, and kicking are common disruptive behaviors exhibited by individuals with Alzheimer's disease. Disruptive behaviors often occur when individuals cannot express themselves or when they do not understand a task they are required to perform. The following learning activities can be used by music therapists in implementing music interventions to decrease disruptive behaviors in individuals with Alzheimer's disease.

Clinical Application 1.5

Target Behavior: Increased movement and flexibility

Music: Recorded instrumental music with a steady, moderate tempo and chosen from a variety of genres and time periods; specifically, songs popular during the individual's teenage to young adult years (see Movement Exercise song recommendations).

Level 1—General Staff

Directions: Choose several different rhythmic songs from CDs or MP3 files to use in a rhythmic instrument playing activity. Hand out rhythm instruments, taking into consideration each individual's use of either both hands or one hand. Play songs while encouraging participants to play their instruments.

Level 2—Volunteer Musician

Directions: Choose several different rhythmic songs from your repertoire and lead a rhythmic instrument playing activity. Make sure each group participant has a rhythm instrument that will be functional for him/her, taking into consideration each individual's use of either both hands or one hand. Before playing each song, demonstrate to group members a few different appropriate rhythmic patterns that would fit into the song.

Level 3—Board-Certified Music Therapist

Activity Name: "Exercise Movement"

Other Goals Addressed: Fine Motor Maintenance, Gross Motor Maintenance, Increased Attention to Task, Increased Mobility, Purposeful Participation. (This activity uses the incompatible response theory to address disruptive behaviors. If participants are actively engaged in this highly structured movement activity, a disruptive response will be less likely to occur.)

Directions: Following recommendations made by Cevasco and Grant (2003), recorded instrumental music (without vocals/singing) should be used when leading movement exercises. Before beginning the activity, make sure each participant is positioned to be able to see your modeled exercise movements. The participants and you should be sitting upright in chairs with support; not in a reclined position. Give each participant a rhythmic instrument to play during the exercises, such as claves, a hand drum with a mallet, or a shaker. Lead the group through movement sequences that are 8 to 16 bars in length. Pair verbal instructions with the physical modeling of each movement throughout the entire activity. Chaining can be used as well to increase success of correct movements. Offer modified movements for individuals with limited mobility.

Clinical Application 1.6

Target Behavior: Increased engagement to task

Music: Chosen from a variety of genres and time periods; specifically, songs that were popular during the individual's teenage to young adult years. Selected songs should tell a story through lyrics and music.

Level 1—General Staff

Directions: Choose several different songs from CDs or MP3 files that tell a story. Hand out rhythm instruments, taking into consideration each individual's use of either both hands or one hand. Play songs while encouraging instrument play. In between each song, lead a short discussion about the song while engaging as many group participants as possible in the discussion. If a disruptive behavior occurs, immediately shift from discussion into playing the song to help distract the frustrated individual.

Level 2—Volunteer Musician

Directions: Lead a "Music Appreciation Performance" by choosing several songs from your repertoire that tell a story. The stories can be about what influenced the composer to create the song, world events happening around the time the song was written or made popular, interesting information about the composer or performer, etc. In between each song, lead a short discussion about the song while engaging as many group participants as possible in the discussion. If a disruptive behavior occurs, immediately shift from discussion into playing the song to help distract the frustrated individual.

Level 3—Board-Certified Music Therapist

Activity Name: "Music Wheel"

Other Goals Addressed: Fine Motor Functioning, Following Directions, Increased Autonomy, Purposeful Participation, Socialization. (This activity uses the incompatible response theory to address disruptive behaviors. If participants are actively engaged in this structured activity with very little "down time" between songs, a disruptive response will be less likely to occur.)

Directions: Create a song genre wheel from foam board or other durable material. Divide the circle into equal sections using different colors. Write the name of a song genre on each section of the wheel. For increased durability, cover the top with clear contact paper. Attach a spinner to the middle of the wheel with nuts and bolts. Ask each group participant to take turns spinning the wheel to determine the genre to be played. As the group progresses, assess each individual's behavioral responses to determine how much time should be spent on each song and on each person's turn spinning the wheel. If precursory disruptive behaviors are recognized, structure the activity to minimize the client's frustration and engage him/her in the music activity.

Clinical Application 1.7

Target Behavior: Increased engagement to task

Music: Chosen from a variety of genres and time periods; specifically, songs that were popular during the individual's teenage to young adult years.

Level 1—General Staff

Directions: Choose several different rhythmic songs from CDs or MP3 files to use in an instrument playing activity. Hand out drums, taking into consideration each individual's use of either both hands or one hand. Play recordings while encouraging participants to play along with their instruments.

Level 2—Volunteer Musician

Directions: Give each group participant a drum appropriate for his/her mobility level. Choose songs from your repertoire that lend themselves to drum accompaniment. Play through the songs, encouraging all group members to find a beat that goes well with the rhythm of the song.

Level 3—Board-Certified Music Therapist

Activity Name: "Therapeutic Drumming"

Other Goals Addressed: Cognitive Stimulation through Improved Short-term Memory and Improved Sequencing, Fine Motor Maintenance, Purposeful Participation, Reality Orientation, Socialization. (This activity uses the incompatible response theory to address disruptive behaviors. If participants are actively engaged in this highly engaging and structured rhythmic activity, a disruptive response will be less likely to occur.)

Directions: Give each group participant a drum appropriate for each individual's ability level. Adaptive drums should be used for individuals with impairments. Then lead the group in a therapeutic drumming activity, focusing on groupings of repeated rhythmic patterns. Participants will be more successful imitating rhythmic patterns if you use eighth note patterns with a cappella singing only (Cevasco & Grant, 2006). To offer more socialization and cognitive stimulation opportunities, ask high functioning participants to demonstrate rhythms for the group to imitate.

Clinical Application 1.8

Target Behavior: Socialization

Music: Chosen from a variety of genres and time periods; specifically, songs that were popular during the individual's teenage to young adult years.

Level 1—General Staff

Directions: Create a Bingo game board from a large piece of foam board. Label ping-pong balls with numbers corresponding to the game board. Pair songs (or several choices of different songs) with each number on the board. Have group participants take turns drawing a ball out of the basket. For a fast-paced activity, play the corresponding song as soon as the ball is drawn. A CD player with multiple CDs loaded will decrease the down-time between songs.

Level 2—Volunteer Musician

Directions: Create a Bingo game board from a large piece of foam board. Label ping-pong balls with numbers corresponding to the game board. Pair songs (or several choices of different songs) with each number on the board. Have group participants take turns drawing a ball out of the basket. For a fast-paced activity, play the corresponding song as soon as the ball is drawn.

Level 3—Board-Certified Music Therapist

Activity Name: "Music BINGO"

Other Goals Addressed: Cognitive Stimulation through Improved Short-term Memory and Improved Sequencing, Fine Motor Maintenance, Purposeful Participation, Reality Orientation, Reminiscence. (This activity uses the incompatible response theory to address disruptive behaviors. If participants are actively engaged in this structured activity with very little "down time" between songs, a disruptive response will be less likely to occur.)

Directions: Create a Bingo game board from a large piece of foam board. Label ping-pong balls with numbers corresponding to the game board. Pair songs (or several choices of different songs) with each number on the board. Have group participants take turns drawing a ball out of the basket. For a fast-paced activity, sing (with live accompaniment) the chosen song as soon as the ball is drawn. To offer more socialization and cognitive stimulation opportunities, ask participants to answer questions and solve clues to determine the song before marking the number on the game board. As the group progresses, assess each individual's behavioral responses to determine how much time should be spent on each song and on each person's turn choosing the bingo ball. If precursory disruptive behaviors are recognized, structure the activity to minimize the individual's frustration and engage the patient in the music activity.

FOCUS AREA 3: ADDRESSING EMOTIONAL NEEDS WITH MUSIC

A diagnosis of probable Alzheimer's disease can be devastating to an individual—especially in the early stages of the illness when cognitive declines begin to occur. As the disease progresses, individuals may transition to long-term care facilities because of an increase in their care needs (Brotons, Koger, & Pickett-Cooper, 1997). Emotional problems may arise for individuals with Alzheimer's disease as a result of changes in their living environment and declines that occur with the illness. The following learning activities illustrate how music can be applied therapeutically to address common emotional problems such as apathy, anxiety, and symptoms of depression.

Clinical Application 1.9

Target Behavior: Increased coping with illness

Music: Chosen from a variety of genres and time periods; specifically, songs that were popular during the individual's teenage to young adult years. Selected songs should incorporate the theme "good things in life" (see Emotion song recommendations).

Level 1—General Staff

Directions: Choose several different songs from CDs or MP3 files that relate to the theme "good things in life," such as "What a Wonderful World," "My Favorite Things," or "I Could Have Danced All Night." Play songs while encouraging participants to discuss the good things in their lives.

Level 2—Volunteer Musician

Directions: Make a performance list from your repertoire of songs that relate to the theme "good things in life," such as "What a Wonderful World," "My Favorite Things," or "I Could Have Danced All Night." Play songs while encouraging participants to discuss the good things in their lives.

Level 3—Board-Certified Music Therapist

Activity Name: "Life Is Good Songwriting"

Other Goals Addressed: Decreased Depression, Decreased Anxiety, Purposeful Participation, Reminiscence, Socialization

Directions: Choose a song with thematic content about "the good things in life," such as "My Favorite Things" or "Glory, Glory, Hallelujah." Encourage each group member to participate in creating a group song that identifies the good things about life. For smaller groups, each group member can create an entire verse, while larger groups will most likely share ideas that will combine into verses. Assess emotional states and coping skill levels for group participants and lead the group discussion accordingly. Pair individuals with weak coping skills with group members with strong coping skills during the group discussion time.

Clinical Application 1.10

Target Behavior: Decreased depression

Music: Chosen from a variety of genres and time periods; specifically, songs that were popular during the individual's teenage to young adult years. Selected songs should include psychosocial themes such as "feeling down," depressed, or lonely (see Emotion song recommendations).

Level 1—General Staff

Directions: Choose several different songs from CDs or MP3 files that have themes relating to feeling down, such as "I'm So Lonesome I Could Cry," "One for My Baby," or "Pass Me Not." Play songs while encouraging participants to discuss their feelings as they relate to the themes expressed in the songs.

Level 2—Volunteer Musician

Directions: Make a performance list from your repertoire of songs that have lyrics about feeling down, such as "I'm So Lonesome I Could Cry," "One for My Baby," or "Pass Me Not." Play songs while encouraging participants to discuss their feelings as they relate to the themes expressed in the songs.

Level 3—Board-Certified Music Therapist

Activity Name: "Lyric Analysis for Depression"

Other Goals Addressed: Decreased Anxiety, Increased Coping Skills, Purposeful Participation, Reminiscence, Socialization

Directions: Choose a song with content about feeling depressed or lonely, such as "I'm So Lonesome I Could Cry," "One for My Baby," or "Pass Me Not." Lead a lyric analysis of the selected songs, focusing on coping strategies for the areas of need that were communicated by the group. Assess emotional states and coping skill levels for group participants and lead the group discussion accordingly. Pair individuals with weak coping skills with group members with strong coping skills during the group discussion time.

Clinical Application 1.11

Target Behavior: Decreased apathy/Increasing will to live

Music: Chosen from a variety of genres and time periods; specifically, songs that were popular during the individual's teenage to young adult years. Selected songs should incorporate the theme "having a purpose in life" (see Emotion song recommendations).

Level 1—General Staff

Directions: Choose several different songs from CDs or MP3 files that have themes relating to having a purpose in life, such as "Young At Heart," "You Light Up My Life," or "His Eye Is on the Sparrow." Play songs while encouraging participants to discuss how they relate to the sentiments expressed in the songs.

Level 2—Volunteer Musician

Directions: Make a performance list from your repertoire of songs that have lyrics relating to having a purpose in life, such as "Young At Heart," "You Light Up My Life," or "His Eye Is on the Sparrow." Play songs while encouraging participants to discuss how they relate to the sentiments expressed in the songs.

Level 3—Board-Certified Music Therapist

Activity Name: "Songwriting for Apathy"

Other Goals Addressed: Decreased Anxiety, Increased Coping Skills, Purposeful Participation, Reminiscence, Socialization

Directions: Choose songs with thematic content relating to having purpose in life, such as "Young At Heart," "You Light Up My Life," or "His Eye Is on the Sparrow." Encourage each group member to participate in creating a group song that identifies the good things about life. For smaller groups, each group member can create an entire verse, while larger groups will most likely share ideas that will combine into verses. Assess emotional states and coping skill levels for group participants and lead the group discussion accordingly. Pair individuals with weak coping skills with group members with strong coping skills during the group discussion time.

Clinical Application 1.12

Target Behavior: Decreased anxiety

Music: Chosen from a variety of genres and time periods; specifically, songs that were popular during the individual's teenage to young adult years. Selected songs should include varying tempos and intensities.

Level 1—General Staff

Directions: Choose several different songs from CDs or MP3 files that have varying tempos and intensities. Start with the songs having the fastest tempos and greatest intensity. As you progress through playing the songs, choose songs that have less intensity and slower tempos so that you end with a song having a very slow tempo and low intensity. This process should take approximately 30 minutes. Group participants may play rhythm instruments with the songs, if desired.

Level 2—Volunteer Musician

Directions: Choose several different songs from your repertoire that have varying tempos and intensities. Start with the songs having the fastest tempos and greatest intensity. As you progress through playing the songs, choose songs that have less intensity and slower tempos so that you end with a song having a very slow tempo and low intensity. This process should take approximately 30 minutes. Group participants may play rhythm instruments with the songs, if desired.

Level 3—Board-Certified Music Therapist

Activity Name: "Iso-Principle for Anxiety"

Other Goals Addressed: Decreased Anxiety, Increased Coping Skills, Purposeful Participation, Reminiscence, Socialization

Directions: Choose songs with varying tempos and intensities. Using the Iso-Principle, match the emotional state of the most anxious person in the group. Using live singing and accompaniment, slowly decrease the intensity and tempo of the music to entrain the anxious participant's emotional state. If the anxious individual displays an increase in anxiety after showing calmer behavior, match the emotional state again and repeat the process. While the length of this process does vary for each person, typically an individual can experience a lasting, calm emotional state within 30–45 minutes. Assess individual emotional states and coping skill levels for group participants and lead any needed group discussion accordingly.

FOCUS AREA 4: ADDRESSING FAMILY/CAREGIVER NEEDS WITH MUSIC

The relationship between a caregiver and loved one suffering from Alzheimer's disease can become strained as the illness progresses. This strain often leads to caregiver burden and stress. Music therapy interventions can be used to decrease caregiver stress and improve the relationship between caregiver and care receiver (Clair, 2002; Clair & Ebberts, 1997). The following learning activities illustrate how caregivers can use music to improve their loved one's orientation to the environment and increase their compliance with activities of daily life.

Clinical Application 1.13

Target Behavior: Increased bonding and connection

Music: Recorded dance music chosen from a variety of genres and time periods; specifically, songs that were popular during the individual's teenage to young adult years.

Level 1—General Staff

Directions: Choose recorded dance music from CDs or MP3 files that was popular during group participants' teenage and young adult years. If possible, schedule the group to accommodate loved ones' visits. Ask for volunteers who might want to dance together. If loved ones are visiting, encourage them to lead their partner in a dance. For individuals who do not have a family member/caregiver present, ask if they would like to dance with another group member.

Level 2—Volunteer Musician

Directions: Choose several different songs from your repertoire that were popular dancing songs during group participants' teenage and young adult years. If possible, schedule the group to accommodate loved ones' visits. Ask for volunteers who might want to dance together. If loved ones are visiting, encourage them to lead their partner in a dance. For individuals who do not have a family member/caregiver present, ask if they would like to dance with another group member.

Level 3—Board-Certified Music Therapist

Activity Name: "Dancing Memories"

Other Goals Addressed: Reminiscence, Quality of Life, Socialization, Increased Sense of Self

Directions: Set up family/caregiver interviews to discover favorite songs shared with their loved one. For spouses, identify favorite songs from memorable occasions, such as songs they danced to while courting or at their wedding. For other family members, identify songs that were the loved ones' favorites from their teenage or young adult years, or songs that are important to their relationship. Schedule a time, either weekly or monthly, for loved ones to come to a dance at your facility. Refer to the individualized song lists when family members attend the dance to provide family members/caregivers opportunities for bonding and reminiscence.

Clinical Application 1.14

Target Behavior: Increased bonding and connection

Music: Recorded dance music chosen from a variety of genres and time periods; specifically, songs that were popular during the individual's teenage to young adult years.

Level 1—General Staff

Directions: Choose several different songs from CDs or MP3 files that relate a story. After gathering individuals in the room for a group interaction time, hand out rhythmic instruments, taking into consideration each individual's use of either both hands or one hand. Play songs while encouraging participants to play their instruments. In between each song, lead a short discussion about the song while engaging as many group participants as possible in the discussion. Encourage family members to sing along and reminisce with their loved ones.

Level 2—Volunteer Musician

Directions: Invite family members/caregivers to attend a "Music Appreciation Performance." Choose several songs from your repertoire that tell a story. These stories can be about what influenced the composer to create the song, world events happening around the time the song was written or made popular, interesting information about the composer or performer, etc. In between each song, lead a short discussion about the song while engaging as many group participants as possible in the discussion. Encourage family members to sing along and reminisce with their loved ones.

Level 3—Board-Certified Music Therapist

Activity Name: "Making Music Together"

Other Goals Addressed: Decreased Anxiety, Reminiscence, Socialization

Directions: Invite family members/caregivers to attend a music session with their loved one. Hand out rhythm instruments for group participants to play along with songs that are sung. If any family members/caregivers are musicians, invite them to play songs during the session, if desired. Allow each family member/caregiver and loved one the opportunity to play the accompaniment of a song on an instrument such as a Q-Chord or autoharp or strum the guitar as you change chords. While each pair is creating music together, encourage eye contact between the pairs as well as hand holding or tapping to the music, where appropriate.

Clinical Application 1.15

Target Behavior: Increased coping skills

Music: Chosen from a variety of genres and time periods; specifically, songs that were popular during the individual's teenage to young adult years. Selected songs should incorporate the theme "the good things in life" (see Emotion song recommendations).

Level 1—General Staff

Directions: Choose several different songs from CDs or MP3 files that have themes relating to the good things in life, such as "What a Wonderful World," "My Favorite Things," or "I Could Have Danced All Night." Invite family members/caregivers to attend a group music session with their loved one. Play songs while encouraging family members/caregivers and their loved ones to discuss the good things in their lives.

Level 2—Volunteer Musician

Directions: Make a performance list from your repertoire of songs that have lyrics about the good things in life, such as "What a Wonderful World," "My Favorite Things," or "I Could Have Danced All Night." Invite family members/caregivers to attend a group music session with their loved ones. Play songs while encouraging family members/caregivers and their loved ones to discuss the good things in their lives.

Level 3—Board-Certified Music Therapist

Activity Name: "Singing and Reflecting"

Other Goals Addressed: Decreased Anxiety, Increased Coping Skills, Increased Problem Solving, Reminiscence, Socialization

Directions: Choose a song with thematic content about good things in life, such as "My Favorite Things" or "Glory, Glory, Hallelujah." Invite family members/caregivers to attend a group music session with their loved ones. Encourage each group member to participate in creating a group song that identifies the good things about life. For smaller groups, each group member can create an entire verse, while larger groups will most likely share ideas that will combine into verses. Assess emotional states and coping skill levels for group participants and lead the group discussion accordingly. Pair individuals with weak coping skills with group members with strong coping skills during the group discussion time.

Clinical Application 1.16

Target Behavior: Increased life satisfaction and rejuvenation

Music: Chosen from a variety of genres and time periods; specifically, songs that were popular during the individual's teenage to young adult years. Selected songs should include notable themes that could represent people in the group (see Thematic song recommendations).

Level 1—General Staff

Directions: Choose several different songs from CDs or MP3 files that have lyrics incorporating themes such as dancing, feeling happy, cars, military service, etc. Invite family members/caregivers to attend a group music time with their loved ones. After each song is played, have group members discuss which member of the group the song reminds them of and explain why. Encourage reminiscence from family members/caregivers about their loved ones' lives and memories evoked by the music.

Level 2—Volunteer Musician

Directions: Make a performance list from your repertoire of songs that have lyrics including themes such as dancing, feeling happy, cars, military service, etc. Invite family members/caregivers to attend a group music time with their loved ones. After each song is played, have group members discuss who among the group that song reminds them of and why. Encourage reminiscence from family members/caregivers about their loved ones' lives and memories evoked by the music.

Level 3—Board-Certified Music Therapist

Activity Name: "Music-Assisted Life Review"

Other Goals Addressed: Increased Coping Skills, Increased Bonding, Reminiscence, Socialization

Directions: Set up interviews with family members/caregivers to find out important life events, personality traits, and meaningful memories for their loved ones. Also find out which style/genre of music their loved one most enjoys. Write songs for each individual that describe and honor their lives. Use the genre style preferred by each individual. Songs can be composed originally or can be written as parodies using existing melodies. Set up either a group time or individual sessions with family members/caregivers to play the songs that were composed. These songs can also be recorded and given to family members/caregivers as a lasting gift.

THEMATIC SONG LISTS

Reminiscence

Accentuate the Positive – Bing Crosby

Ain't Misbehavin' – Ella Fitzgerald

Ain't No Mountain High Enough – Marvin Gaye

Always on My Mind – Willie Nelson

America (My Country 'Tis of Thee) – Samuel Francis Smith

America, the Beautiful – Samuel Ward

At Last – Ella Fitzgerald

Baby Love – The Supremes

Beautiful Dreamer – Stephen Foster

Bewitched, Bothered, and Bewildered – Ella Fitzgerald, etc.

Blue – Patsy Cline / Leanne Rimes

Blue Eyes Cryin' in the Rain – Willie Nelson

Blueberry Hill – Fats Domino

Boogie Woogie Bugle Boy – Andrews Sisters

Brown Eyed Girl – Van Morrison

By the Light of the Silvery Moon – Gus Edwards

Can't Help Falling in Love – Elvis Presley

Catch a Falling Star – Perry Como

Chattanooga Choo Choo – Glenn Miller

Climb Every Mountain – Sound of Music

Come Fly With Me – Frank Sinatra

Could I Have This Dance – Anne Murray

Crazy – Patsy Cline

Daisy Bell (Bicycle Built for Two) – Harry Dacre

Danny Boy – Frederick Weatherly

Dock of the Bay – Otis Redding

Don't Get Around Much Anymore – Duke Ellington

Dream, Dream, Dream – Everly Brothers

Earth Angel – Buddy Holly

Edelweiss – The Sound of Music

Five Foot Two – Dean Martin

Fly Me to the Moon – Frank Sinatra

The Gambler – Kenny Rogers

Georgia on My Mind – Willie Nelson

Getting to Know You – The King and I

Give My Regards to Broadway – George Cohan

God Bless America – Irving Berlin

Goody Goody – Ella Fitzgerald

Greensleeves

Happy Together – Bonner/Gordon

Hello Darlin' – Conway Twitty

Hey, Good Lookin' – Hank Williams

Home on the Range – Roy Rogers

Honky Tonk Blues – Hank Williams

I Could Have Danced All Night – My Fair Lady

I Fall to Pieces – Patsy Cline

I Got Rhythm – George Gershwin

I Got You – James Brown

I Heard It Through the Grapevine – Marvin Gaye

I Say a Little Prayer for You – Dionne Warwick

I Walk the Line – Johnny Cash

I'm Forever Blowing Bubbles – The Passing Show

I'm So Lonesome I Could Cry – Hank Williams

I've Been Working on the Railroad – Sandhills Sixteen

The Impossible Dream – Man of La Mancha

In the Good Old Summertime – Connie Francis

In the Still of the Night – The Five Satins

It Had to Be You – Frank Sinatra

It's Only a Paper Moon – Ella Fitzgerald

It's Only Make Believe – Conway Twitty

Jolene – Dolly Parton

King of the Road – Roger Miller

Let Me Call You Sweetheart – Bing Crosby

L-O-V-E ("L" is for the way you look at me) – Nat King Cole

Lucille – Kenny Rogers

Matchmaker – Fiddler on the Roof

Memory – Cats

Moon River – Johnny Mercer

Move It on Over – Hank Williams

My Bonnie Lies Over the Ocean

My Favorite Things – The Sound of Music

My Girl – The Temptations

My Guy – Mary Wells

My Way – Frank Sinatra

My Wild Irish Rose – Chauncey Olcott

Oh, Susanna – Stephen Foster

Oh, What a Beautiful Morning – Oklahoma

Oklahoma! – Oklahoma

Old Folks at Home (Swanee River) – Stephen Foster

On the Road Again – Willie Nelson

Over the Rainbow – The Wizard of Oz

Put on a Happy Face – Bye Bye, Birdie

Rocky Top – Lynn Anderson

Sentimental Journey – Doris Day

Seventy-six Trombones – Music Man

Singin' in the Rain – Singin' in the Rain

Some Enchanted Evening – South Pacific

Someone to Watch Over Me – Ella Fitzgerald

Splish Splash – Bobby Darin

Stand by Me – Temptations / Ben E. King

Stand by Your Man – Tammy Wynette

Star Spangled Banner

Strangers in the Night – Frank Sinatra

Summertime – Ella Fitzgerald

Sunrise, Sunset – Fiddler on the Roof

Surrey with the Fringe on Top – Oklahoma!

Suspicious Minds – Elvis Presley

Swingin' – John Anderson

Swingin' on a Star – Bing Crosby

Take These Chains – Hank Williams

Tennessee Waltz – Anne Murray

They Can't Take That Away From Me – Frank Sinatra

Through the Years – Kenny Rogers

Till There Was You – Music Man

To All the Girls I've Loved Before – Willie Nelson

Try to Remember – The Fantasticks

The Twist – Chubby Checker

Unchained Melody – Righteous Brothers

Under the Boardwalk – The Drifters

Unforgettable – Nat King Cole

Walkin' After Midnight – Patsy Cline

The Way You Do the Thing You Do – Temptations

When a Man Loves a Woman – Percy Sledge

Wonderful World – Louis Armstrong

Wouldn't It Be Loverly – My Fair Lady

You Are My Sunshine – Oliver Hood

You Decorated My Life – Kenny Rogers

You Needed Me – Anne Murray

Young at Heart – Frank Sinatra

Your Cheatin' Heart – Hank Williams

Songs That Can Represent People

Boogie Woogie Bugle Boy – Andrews Sisters

Chattanooga Choo Choo – Glenn Miller

Come Fly With Me – Frank Sinatra

Danny Boy – Frederick Weatherly

Dock of the Bay – Otis Redding

Don't Get Around Much Anymore – Duke Ellington

Five Foot Two – Dean Martin

The Gambler – Kenny Rogers

Georgia on My Mind – Willie Nelson

Give My Regards to Broadway – Judy Garland

Home on the Range – Roy Rogers

I Could Have Danced All Night – My Fair Lady

I Walk the Line – Johnny Cash

The Impossible Dream – Man of La Mancha

King of the Road – Roger Miller

My Girl – The Temptations

My Guy – Mary Wells

My Way – Frank Sinatra

On the Road Again – Willie Nelson

Rocky Top – Lynn Anderson

Stand by Me – Temptations / Ben E. King

Stand by Your Man – Tammy Wynette

Strangers in the Night – Frank Sinatra

Till There Was You – Music Man

To All the Girls I've Loved Before – Willie Nelson

Try to Remember – The Fantasticks

Under the Boardwalk – The Drifters

The Way You Do the Thing You Do – Temptations

When a Man Loves a Woman – Percy Sledge

Wouldn't It Be Loverly – My Fair Lady

You Are My Sunshine – Oliver Hood

Songs with Emotion Content

▪ *Feeling Down*

Blue – Patsy Cline / Leanne Rimes

Blue Eyes Cryin' in the Rain – Willie Nelson

Crazy – Patsy Cline

Don't Get Around Much Anymore – Duke Ellington

Everyday I Have the Blues – Count Basie

I Fall to Pieces – Patsy Cline

I'm So Lonesome I Could Cry – Hank Williams

The Impossible Dream – Man of La Mancha

Jolene – Dolly Parton

Lucille – Kenny Rogers

Memory – Cats

One for My Baby – Frank Sinatra

Pass Me Not – Hymn

Precious Lord – Hymn

Sentimental Journey – Doris Day

Suspicious Minds – Elvis Presley

Take These Chains – Hank Williams

Your Cheatin' Heart – Hank Williams

▪ *Good Things / Purpose in Life*

Accentuate the Positive – Bing Crosby and the Andrews Sisters

Amazing Grace – Hymn

Because He Lives – Hymn

Glory, Glory Hallelujah – Hymn

Happy Together – Bonner/Gordon

I Could Have Danced All Night – My Fair Lady

I Have Decided to Follow Jesus – Hymn

I Say a Little Prayer for You – Dionne Warwick

It is Well with My Soul – Hymn

My Favorite Things – Sound of Music

Oh, What a Beautiful Morning – Oklahoma

Put on a Happy Face – Bye Bye, Birdie

What a Wonderful World – Louis Armstrong

You Needed Me – Anne Murray

Songs for Movement Exercises (instrumental versions recommended)

Back Bay Shuffle – Artie Shaw
Boogie Woogie – Tommy Dorsey
Bumble Boogie – Freddie Martin
Casa Loma Stomp – Glen Gray
Chattanooga Choo Choo – Glenn Miller
Cherokee – Charlie Barnet
Cotton Tail – Duke Ellington
In the Mood – Glenn Miller
It Don't Mean a Thing – Duke Ellington

King Porter Stomp – Benny Goodman
Sing, Sing, Sing – Benny Goodman
Stompin' at the Savoy – Benny Goodman
String of Pearls – Glenn Miller
Sweet Georgia Brown – Ella Fitzgerald
Take the "A" Train – Duke Ellington
Tangerine – Jimmy Dorsey
Tuxedo Junction – Erskine Hawkins

REFERENCES

Brotons, M., & Koger, S. M. (2000). The impact of music therapy on language functioning in dementia. *Journal of Music Therapy, 37*(3), 183–195.

Brotons, M., Koger, S. M., & Pickett-Cooper, P. (1997). Music and dementias: A review of literature. *Journal of Music Therapy, 34*, 204–245.

Carruth, E. K. (1997). The effects of singing and the spaced retrieval technique on improving face-name recognition in nursing home residents with memory loss. *Journal of Music Therapy, 34*(3), 165–186.

Cevasco, A. M., & Grant, R. E. (2003). Comparison of different methods for eliciting exercise-to-music for clients with Alzheimer's disease. *Journal of Music Therapy, 40*(1), 41–56.

Cevasco, A. M., & Grant, R. E. (2006). Value of musical instruments used by the therapist to elicit responses from individuals in various stages of Alzheimer's disease. *Journal of Music Therapy, 43*, 226–246.

Clair, A. A. (2002). The effects of music therapy on engagement in family caregiver and care receiver couples with dementia. *American Journal of Alzheimer's Disease and Other Dementias, 17*(5), 286-290.

Clair, A. A., & Ebberts, A. G. (1997). The effects of music therapy on interactions between family caregivers and their care receivers with late stage dementia. *Journal of Music Therapy, 34*(3), 148–164.

Prickett, C. A., & Moore, R. S. (1991). The use of music to aid memory of Alzheimer's patients. *Journal of Music Therapy, 28*(2), 101–110.

Smith, G. (1986). A comparison of the effects of three treatment interventions on cognitive functioning of Alzheimer patients. *Music Therapy, 6A*(1), 41–56.

UNIT II
MUSIC THERAPY IN HOSPICE
AND
PALLIATIVE CARE

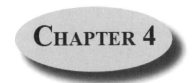

CHAPTER 4

INTRODUCTION TO HOSPICE AND PALLIATIVE CARE AND MUSIC THERAPY

That song is "our song" and I know he hears you playing it, even though he can't tell us that right now. —Mrs. P. (wife of hospice patient)

I wish you could come see me every day. Music days are my best days. —Ms. K.

THE HOSPICE MOVEMENT

The hospice movement has been one of the most influential factors in the fields of grief, death, and dying (Hilliard, 2005a; Rando, 1984; Worden, 2009). A hospice can be defined as a program of palliative and supportive services that provides physical, psychological, social, and spiritual care for dying persons and their families (National Hospice Organization, 1981, as cited in Rando, 1984, p. 296). Hospice care is usually available in private homes, nursing homes, assisted living facilities, hospitals, and hospice inpatient facilities. Hospice organizations believe that death is a normal life process that should be neither hastened nor postponed (Rando, 1984). The philosophy of hospice care is to affirm life and to allow patients to experience the best quality of life possible during the time they have remaining (Hilliard, 2005a; Rando, 1984).

The hospice mission also includes providing support to the families of dying patients, both during the patient's care and after the death. Hospice organizations recognize that a terminal illness affects not only the patient, but also the entire family. Roles and routines often change when one family member becomes too sick to maintain his or her usual level of participation in running the household. In addition to providing care for the patient, the hospice team can assist the family in keeping the household running smoothly. Hospice volunteers can be assigned to help with childcare, pet care, and simple household chores. Hospice social workers assist the family with financial planning, medical paperwork, nursing home placement, or funeral preparation. Hospice bereavement counselors also follow each family for 1 year after the death and provide individual and group counseling to the community at large. Research has shown that participation in a comprehensive hospice program is associated with better grief resolution outcomes for family members than for those whose loved ones died in a hospital without hospice care (Ransford & Smith, 1991; Smith, 1984).

The hospice movement has a grassroots element and is usually community-based and largely staffed by volunteers. Kübler-Ross was a strong promoter of the hospice movement in the 1970s and urged medical professionals to improve focus on treating symptoms and providing comfort to dying patients (Rando, 1984). By 1985 there were over 800 hospices nationwide, specific accreditation requirements, and the beginnings of Medicare and Medicaid reimbursement. Today there are over 3,300 hospices operating in the United States, staffed by both full- and part-time paid employees (Hilliard, 2005a).

One of the biggest misconceptions about hospice is that "it's where you go to die." Patients and families are often reluctant to begin hospice services because they feel they are "giving up" or simply waiting for the patient to die. Even doctors are often reluctant to refer for hospice care until the last minute because their training has focused them on finding and curing the problem rather than palliating symptoms (Rando, 1984). Hospice organizations usually have community relations staff and referral specialists who spend time providing continued education in the community and in doctors' offices about the benefits of hospice care. Calling in hospice does not mean the patient is about to die; it means that aggressive or curative treatments are no longer indicated. The hospice team designs a plan of care for optimal symptom management and quality of life for each patient. In fact, the earlier the hospice referral is made, the longer the patient and family will have the benefit of the physical care and emotional support of the hospice team. Too often, the patient is referred in the last week of life when uncontrolled pain and terminal agitation are the focus of care until the patient's death. These situations afford little time for the hospice team to get the patient comfortable or to prepare the family emotionally for the experience.

The typical hospice referral is made when a clinician determines that a patient has 6 months or less to live; however, patients often remain in the program longer if evaluations show a continual steady decline in health. It is not unheard of for an individual to be a hospice patient for 2 to 3 years, especially in those disease processes with a slow progression. In these cases, the hospice team, the patient, and the patient's family form strong bonds that can ease the burden of the terminal illness. Conversely, those hospice patients who do not decline or who show improvement in health and functioning will be discharged from the hospice program with the option to be readmitted if disease progression resumes. Ironically, hospice patients and families often become so accustomed to the benefits of the hospice team that they can be upset when the patient is discharged, even though this means that the patient's health has improved.

Hospice organizations are structured as an interdisciplinary team (IDT) of staff members, all working toward the same goals for each patient (Speck, 2006). This unique team approach provides hospice staff with opportunities for collaboration, growth, and success. According to the Medicare Hospice Benefit of 1983, federal law requires hospices to structure their meetings in an IDT format (Wittenberg-Lyles, Oliver, Demiris, & Courtney, 2007). A survey of hospice agencies revealed a variation among the types of disciplines participating in IDT meetings (Wittenberg-Lyles et al., 2007); however, Medicare mandates that the IDT include a doctor, nurse, social worker, chaplain, and volunteers (Kovacs & Bronstein, 1999; Wittenberg-Lyles et al., 2007). Additional members of the team not required by Medicare may include occupational therapists, art therapists, music therapists, home health aides, and bereavement counselors. Figure 1 illustrates the organizational structure of the IDT. The patient and the patient's family are the focus of the team and the IDT members are equal around the table, working together toward the same general goals.

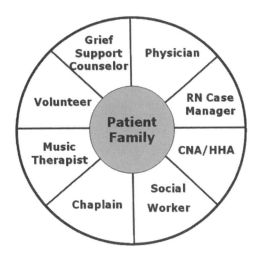

Figure 1: The Interdisciplinary Team

The average IDT meeting is held either weekly or biweekly, lasts approximately 1 to 2 hours, and usually involves 10 to 20 people (Wittenberg-Lyles et al., 2007). Most hospices report a high level of collaboration between the various disciplines regardless of how many members are on the team (Parker-Oliver, Bronstein, & Kurzejeski, 2005). There are many positive aspects to working in the IDT model, and this teamwork is often considered the hallmark of hospice care. Communication between team members and role blending, defined as overlapping duties between disciplines (Corless & Nicholas, 2004), can lead to improved patient care and problem solving. However, role blending can also lead to vulnerability for IDT members, as each member's work is exposed to other team members' scrutiny. Nonetheless, most research in this area indicates that the IDT approach reduces stress to a greater degree than it increases stress for hospice workers (McNurlen, 1989).

QUALITY OF LIFE

The focus of hospice care is to palliate or manage symptoms rather than cure, and so increased quality of life is the fundamental endpoint (Axelsson & Per-Olow, 1999). The chief mission of hospice care is to assist patients in living out their remaining days in as much comfort as possible and with the highest quality of life possible (Byock, 1998). This mission includes having every member of the IDT work together to reduce each patient's physical symptoms, such as acute and chronic pain, discomfort, anxiety, and nausea. Quality of life in end-of-life care is a multidimensional construct that comprises a wide range of patient needs. Interpersonal relationships, reflections of the past, acceptance and perceptions of the present, and expectations of the future are some of the influences on a patient's perceived quality of life (Steinhauser, 2002). Thus, quality of life may be the most helpful evaluative tool in measuring the effectiveness of palliative care. When dealing with the multidimensional needs of hospice patients, considering the care of the "whole person" is paramount in order to best assist and support the patient and his or her family (Hilliard, 2001). Hospice organizations provide patient care for physical, psychosocial, and spiritual needs and must be flexible to keep up with the ever-changing situation found in each patient.

Hospice patients face an array of multidimensional psychosocial issues during their end-of-life journeys (MacLeod, 2008). Intense emotions, including those described in Kübler-Ross's (1969) Five Stages of Grief, can make it difficult for patients to express themselves and for family members to communicate with one another (Bright, 1986; Hilliard, 2005a; Wlodarczyk, 2009). Hospice organizations are known for utilizing a variety of creative activities and therapies to aid patients and families in self-expression during this difficult time. Of all these creative therapies, music therapy has the largest body of research supporting its effectiveness as an intervention that promotes self-expression and improved communication between hospice patients and caregivers (Bailey, 1984; Clements-Cortés, 2004; Hilliard, 2001, 2005a; Munro, 1984; Nelson, 2006; West, 1994, Wlodarczyk, 2009).

MUSIC THERAPY IN HOSPICE AND PALLIATIVE CARE

The comprehensive body of research with music therapy can be reduced to a few recurring principles: music appeals to almost everyone, music is reinforcing, music evokes memories, and music provides an outlet for self-expression. While providing hospice patients with CDs and a CD player in their rooms can be beneficial, this cannot replicate the personal interaction between a music therapist and a patient. At a time when the patient may be isolated and feeling out of control, a music therapy session can provide a time for socializing, making choices, and expressing feelings in a safe environment. Though music is believed by many to be relaxing, hospice staff members often overlook the type of music being used. Instrumental or "New Age" CDs are frequently distributed to hospice patients as relaxing music, though this type of music may not have the same relaxing effect on everyone. Music therapists are trained to use only patient-preferred music in their sessions, as research has shown that familiar music will achieve the greatest benefit for each patient (Gibbons, 1977; Hilliard, 2005a; Moore, Staum, & Brotons, 1992; O'Callaghan, 2009; Porchet-Munro, 1993; Wlodarczyk, 2009).

Music therapy has become a widely accepted discipline in hospice and palliative care. Over the last three decades, hospice music therapists have benefited from increased job availability and have contributed to a substantial body of research in the field (Hilliard, 2005b; O'Callaghan, 2009). Music therapists have become valued members of the IDT (Wlodarczyk, 2008) and are regularly consulted on care planning and decision making for their patients. The benefits of hospice music therapy have been seen in all facets of patient care—physical, psychosocial, and spiritual (Hilliard, 2005a, 2005b; O'Callaghan, 2009; Wlodarczyk, 2007).

The overall focus of music therapy in hospice and palliative care is to enhance patients' quality of life through the use of live music and personal interaction. Music interventions can be tailored to meet individual patients' physical, emotional, or spiritual needs. Music therapists are trained to reduce patients' perception of pain, to assist patients in working through the stages of grief, and to provide support to patients as they deal with issues of spiritual distress (Hilliard, 2005a). Hilliard (2001) describes the music therapist as a guide on the hospice patient's search for "hope, meaning, and a sense of purpose." Music therapists can collaborate with other IDT members to offer patients a wider range of interventions for maintaining comfort and quality of life.

An increasing body of evidence supports music therapy's inclusion on the IDT as a successful intervention in the hospice setting. Music therapy interventions can be employed to decrease perception of pain and anxiety, reduce depressive symptoms, enhance quality of life, and provide spiritual support (Batzner, 2003; Beck, 1991; Calovini, 1993; Clements-Cortés, 2004; Hilliard, 2003; Krout, 2003; Nguyen, 2003; Wlodarczyk, 2007). Music therapy interventions used with patients and their family members include therapeutic singing, music listening, music-assisted relaxation, life review, and songwriting. There is an abundance of qualitative research describing successful music therapy interventions at the end-of-life, but there is a need for more quantitative research in this area. Since research in end-of-life care raises certain ethical considerations relevant to respect for and privacy of the dying patient, hospice music therapy researchers should remain sensitive when designing appropriate studies for this setting.

Music therapy interventions for hospice patients are often the same as those used with other music therapy clients, but they are tailored to the needs of individuals facing a terminal illness. Music therapy can provide an outlet for hospice patients to express feelings regarding the dying process and can increase opportunities for socialization. Music can also be used as an avenue for personal reflection. Both familiar song lyrics or patient-composed song lyrics can facilitate communication of emotions or messages to loved ones. Songs that were popular during different stages of one's life can also facilitate the review of important events such as births, deaths, weddings, and funerals. Music can also be used with hospice patients to increase relaxation, decrease agitation, and provide emotional support to persons who are experiencing discomfort during their final days. When a hospice patient begins to decline and death is imminent, singing together can also provide a musical structure in which family members can participate in lasting positive interactions with their loved ones, and in doing so, derive a sense of peace and closure (Krout, 2003).

Songwriting and lyric analysis are well researched music therapy interventions that have been effective with hospice patients and their families. These interventions can provide opportunities for self-expression, resolution of difficult relationships, expression of hope for future generations, and a means of saying goodbye (Hilliard, 2005a; Krout, 2005; Nguyen, 2003; O'Callaghan, 1996, 1997, 2009; Whitall, 1991; Wlodarczyk, 2009). Music therapists are skilled at structuring the songwriting process to fit each client's needs and ability level. The process can be as simple as a fill-in-the-blank worksheet or as complex as creating original music and lyrics (Wlodarczyk, 2009). Song lyrics can be expressed as literal thoughts and feelings or in themes and metaphors (Thompson, 2009). Existing patient-preferred songs or songs that patients and their families have written during music therapy sessions can be used in lyric analysis (Hilliard, 2005a; Wlodarczyk, 2009). Music therapists can choose songs with specific thematic content to elicit discussion when patients are reluctant to engage in self-expression (Silverman, 2009; Standley & Jones, 2007).

Individuals facing the end of life often question their ethics, values, and spiritual beliefs (Bright, 1986; Hilliard, 2005a; Wlodarczyk, 2007). Though hospice patients represent a vast spectrum of spiritual and religious backgrounds, the basic need to make sense of life and death is universal. Music therapy can address issues of spiritual distress and provide spiritual comfort through live music-making, lyrics analysis, songwriting, and music-assisted worship, prayer, or meditation (Aldridge, 1995; Foxglove & Tyas, 2000; Hilliard, 2005a; Lipe, 2002; Magill, 2001; O'Callaghan, 2009; Okamoto, 2004; Ryan, 1996; Salmon, 2001; Wlodarczyk, 2007). Music therapists can schedule a joint visit with the hospice chaplain to provide a multisensory experience that "brings church to the patient" when the patient becomes too sick to attend their preferred house of worship.

THE MUSIC THERAPIST AS AN IDT MEMBER

It is important to continue to educate other hospice professionals regarding what music therapy can bring to the IDT because music therapy is a relatively new field and IDT membership frequently changes (Mandel, 1993; Porchet-Munro, 1993). The music therapist, like other IDT members, maintains open and constant communication with the team to ensure that each patient's goals are being met. The music therapist can make observations in his or her visit that will aid other IDT members, such as reporting a patient's pain level or relaying an observed conflict between two family members. The music therapist also completes the same documentation for each visit as the other IDT members. It is important for the music therapist to use this documentation to report any observable decline in functioning from week to week, such as less breath support available for singing, fewer verbalizations made, less strength for grasping an instrument, decreased alertness, etc. These observations help the IDT determine if patients are maintaining the criteria for hospice certification. Similarly, if the music therapist observes that these abilities are improving, then the documentation would support that the patient may be discharged from hospice care.

Spiritual care has been mentioned as an opportunity for collaboration between music therapists and chaplains. Music therapists can support other members of the IDT as well. Joint visits with social workers and volunteers can increase opportunities to engage the patient in life review sessions and create projects that incorporate lasting memories for the family to keep. In instances of acute pain or agitation, music therapists can work to keep patients calm and distracted before medication takes effect, freeing the nurse to see other patients (Curtis, 1986; Gallagher, Lagman, Walsh, Davis, & LeGrand, 2006). Music therapists may also assist with procedural support to distract and relax patients during painful nursing procedures, such as catheter insertion, disimpaction, or a wound dressing change (Kwekkeboom, 2003; Lee, 2005; Longfield, 1995). Music therapists can assist home health aides during bathing and grooming procedures to reduce agitation for patients who are confused. If music therapy can decrease the length of time needed for these procedures and the amount of trauma to the patient, then outcomes will be positive for all involved. Nursing staff may benefit from a more manageable schedule, and patient and family satisfaction with the hospice may improve.

Collaboration with IDT members can continue throughout the entirety of each patient's hospice journey. Music therapists use their unique skill set to enhance the efficacy of each patient's care plan and to contribute to an overall improved quality of life for each patient, whether they are in the hospice program for one week or several years (Abbott, 1995; Hilliard, 2003, 2004b, 2005b; Nelson, 2006). Near the end of a patient's life, the music therapist is often called to ease the suffering at the bedside when death is imminent (Krout, 2003). These intimate music therapy sessions can provide a structure or "safety net" in which family members can participate in a final positive interaction with the patient, saying goodbye and hopefully deriving a sense of closure and peace. The family members may wish to sing songs together that are special to the patient or the family, creating a reverent atmosphere that can be very comforting and peaceful for all present. At this time the music therapist provides support to the IDT as well as the family members gathered at the bedside. Following the death, the music therapist is often asked by the family to sing at the patient's funeral, as a way to honor the patient and assist in bringing closure to the therapeutic relationship (Salmon, 2002; Wlodarczyk, 2007). Collaboration between the music therapist and the chaplain for memorial planning often results in a meaningful celebration of the patient's life that is true to the way the patient wanted to be remembered.

MUSIC THERAPY IN BEREAVEMENT CARE

Typically, the hospice team follows each family for 1 year following the patient's death to assist in the transition and to provide bereavement care for the family. While grief reactions affect the entire person, each individual's response to grief is unique (Worden, 2009). Observable emotional and behavioral grief reactions include crying, withdrawal, distraction, angry outbursts, and forgetfulness. Physical manifestations of grief include loss of appetite or overeating, headaches and body aches, digestive problems, lethargy, and insomnia (Worden, 2009). Spiritual responses range from questioning previously held beliefs to feeling an increased sense of spirituality. Hospice music therapists can work with bereavement counselors to help families process the pain of their loved one's death through a variety of creative interventions.

Reflection is a common practice for those who are grieving. It is natural for the griever to constantly reflect upon memories of the deceased, thoughts about why the death occurred, expectations for the future, and the pain of the loss (Nerken, 1993). Music has been a fundamental component of bereavement rituals throughout history and across cultures (Aborampah, 1999; Amir, 1998; Berger, 2006; Jones, Baker, & Day, 2004). Music that was meaningful to the deceased is typically played or performed at memorial services, funerals, and life celebrations. Planning appropriate music for these rituals can be an important part of the grieving process. Survivors of the deceased often give much consideration to choosing music that both honors the dead and brings comfort to the grieving (Castle & Phillips, 2003; Hayslip, Booher, Scoles, & Guarnaccia, 2007). Active music participation during bereavement rituals, such as singing and dancing, is common in many cultures and may aid the bereaved in expressing their grief (Aborampah, 1999; Amir, 1998; Wexler, 1989). Music can assist the griever in the process of reflection and in achieving grief resolution, the point at which an individual has redefined meaning and purpose in life without the deceased (Augspurger, 1977). It can also help family members to incorporate memories of the deceased into their ongoing lives in a positive manner (Catoe, 1992).

Music therapists can utilize the same interventions with the bereaved as with hospice patients, tailoring them to each individual to address the specific loss. Active music making, such as group drumming, can provide an outlet for the emotional and physical expression of grief. Songwriting can give individuals who are grieving an opportunity to put into song lyrics any sentiments that they did not get a chance to share before their loved one died. Music therapy for persons who are grieving can take place in one-on-one sessions or in a group setting. Because the work with persons who are grieving is so sensitive in nature, there is a lack of music therapy research in the area of bereavement. Still, the research that is available suggests that music therapy can be an effective modality in bereavement, warranting further investigation (Wlodarczyk, 2010).

CONCLUSION

This overview outlines the many benefits of music therapy as a standard of care in the hospice setting. Two modes of evidence that have been at work over the years have helped advance job opportunities for hospice music therapists: the increasing availability of published research, and patient and family reports of satisfaction with music therapy services. Oftentimes research initially is the deciding factor that opens the door for a music therapist; and once hospice administrators hear of the benefits of music therapy from the patients and families being served, new music therapy positions are more likely to be created. Though hospices are made up of caring individuals who want to serve the community, they are still subject to competition like any other business. The addition of a music therapy program can give one local hospice an advantage over another. This can be a powerful selling point for the music therapist who wants to start a new hospice program.

Two consecutive surveys of hospice administrators' knowledge of music therapy revealed that the effectiveness of music therapy in the hospice setting is becoming more well known (Hilliard, 2004a). Ninety-five percent of surveyed hospice administrators were aware of the benefits of music therapy and stated that they had heard about it at conferences and from journal publications. The most frequently cited reason for not hiring a music therapist was insufficient funding (Hilliard, 2004a). Subsequently, there is a need for music therapists to become more familiar with the business aspect of hospice organizations. When music therapists are more knowledgeable in marketing, grant writing, and fundraising, they are more likely to be successful when proposing a new music therapy program to a hospice (Hilliard, 2004a, 2005a).

REFERENCES

Abbott, C. M. (1995). *The effects of music therapy on the perceived quality of life of patients with terminal illness in a hospice setting.* Unpublished master's thesis, Western Michigan University, Kalamazoo.

Aborampah, O. (1999). Women's roles in the mourning rituals of the Akan of Ghana. *Ethnology, 38*(3), 257–271.

Aldridge, D. (1995). Spirituality, hope and music therapy. *The Arts in Psychotherapy, 22*(2), 103–109.

Amir, D. (1998). The use of Israeli folksongs in dealing with women's bereavement and loss in music therapy. In D. Dokter (Ed.), *Arts therapies, refugees and migrants: Reaching across borders* (pp. 217–235). London: Jessica Kingsley.

Augspurger, R. E. (1977). *Grief resolution among recent spouse-bereaved individuals.* Unpublished doctoral dissertation, Northwestern University, Chicago.

Axelsson, B., & Per-Olow, S. (1999). Assessment of quality of life in palliative care: Psychometric properties of a short questionnaire. *Acta Oncologica, 38*(2), 229–237.

Bailey, L. M. (1984). The use of songs in music therapy with cancer patients and their families. *Music Therapy, 4*, 5–17.

Batzner, K. W. (2003). *The effect of therapist vocal improvisation on discomfort behaviors of in-patient hospice clients.* Unpublished master's thesis, University of Kansas, Lawrence.

Beck, S. C. (1991). The therapeutic use of music for cancer-related pain. *Oncology Nursing Forum, 18*(8), 1327–1337.

Berger, J. S. (2006). *Music of the soul: Composing life out of loss.* New York: Routledge/Taylor & Francis Group.

Bright, R. (1986). *Grieving: A handbook for those who care.* St Louis, MO: MMB Music.

Byock, I. (1998). Measuring quality of life for patients with terminal illness: The Missoula-VITAS® Quality of Life Index. *Palliative Medicine, 12,* 231–244.

Calovini, B. S. (1993). *The effect of participation in one music therapy session on state anxiety in hospice patients.* Unpublished master's thesis, Case Western Reserve University, Cleveland, OH.

Castle, J., & Phillips, W. L. (2003). Grief rituals: Aspects that facilitate adjustment to bereavement. *Journal of Loss and Trauma, 8,* 41–71.

Catoe, R. (1992). *The effects of the exposure to death events and grief resolution training on the intensity of bereavement of police officers.* Unpublished doctoral dissertation, University of Maryland, College Park.

Clements-Cortés, A. (2004). The use of music in facilitating emotional expression in the terminally ill. *American Journal of Hospice and Palliative Medicine, 21*(4), 255–260.

Corless, I. B., & Nicholas, P. K. (2004). The interdisciplinary team: An oxymoron? In J. Berzoff & P. R. Silverman (Eds.), *Living with dying: A handbook for end-of-life healthcare practitioners* (pp. 161–170). New York: Columbia University Press.

Curtis, S. L. (1986). The effect of music on pain relief and relaxation of the terminally ill. *Journal of Music Therapy, 23*(1), 10–24.

Foxglove, T., & Tyas, B. (2000). Using music as a spiritual tool in palliative care. *European Journal of Palliative Care, 7*(2), 63–65.

Gallagher, L. M., Lagman, R., Walsh, D., Davis, M. P., & LeGrand, S. B. (2006). The clinical effects of music therapy in palliative medicine. *Supportive Care in Cancer, 14*(8), 859–866.

Gibbons, A. C. (1977). Pop music preferences of elderly persons. *Journal of Music Therapy, 14,* 180–189.

Hayslip, B., Booher, S. K., Scoles, M. T., & Guarnaccia, C. A. (2007). Assessing adults' difficulty in coping with funerals. *Omega, 55*(2), 93–115.

Hilliard, R. E. (2001). The use of music therapy in meeting the multidimensional needs of hospice patients and families. *Journal of Palliative Care, 17*(3), 161–166.

Hilliard, R. E. (2003). The effects of music therapy on quality of life and length of life of hospice patients diagnosed with terminal cancer. *Journal of Music Therapy, 40,* 113–137.

Hilliard, R. E. (2004a). Hospice administrators' knowledge of music therapy: A comparative analysis of surveys. *Music Therapy Perspectives, 22*(2), 104–108.

Hilliard, R. E. (2004b). A post-hoc analysis of music therapy services for residents in nursing homes receiving hospice care. *Journal of Music Therapy, 41,* 266–281.

Hilliard, R. E. (2005a). *Hospice and palliative care music therapy: A guide to program development and clinical care.* Cherry Hill, NJ: Jeffrey Books.

Hilliard, R. E. (2005b). Music therapy in hospice and palliative care: A review of the empirical data. *Evidenced-based Complementary and Alternative Medicine, 2*(2), 173–178.

Jones, C., Baker, F., & Day, T. (2004). From healing rituals to music therapy: Bridging the cultural divide between therapist and young Sudanese refugees. *The Arts in Psychotherapy, 31,* 89–100.

Kovacs, P. J., & Bronstein, L. R. (1999). Preparation for oncology settings: What hospice social workers say they need. *Health & Social Work, 24*(1), 57–64.

Krout, R. (2003). Music therapy with imminently dying hospice patients and their families: Facilitating release near the time of death. *American Journal of Hospice and Palliative Medicine, 20*(2), 129–134.

Krout, R. (2005). Applications of music therapist-composed songs in creating participant connections and facilitating goals and rituals during one-time bereavement support groups and programs. *Music Therapy Perspectives, 23*, 118–128.

Kübler-Ross, E. (1969). *On death and dying.* New York: Macmillan.

Kwekkeboom, K. L. (2003). Music versus distraction for procedural pain and anxiety in patients with cancer. *Oncology Nursing Forum, 30*(3), 433–440.

Lee, H. J. (2005). *The effect of live music via the iso-principle on pain management in palliative care as measured by self-report using a graphic rating scale (GRS) and pulse rate.* Unpublished master's thesis, The Florida State University, Tallahassee.

Lipe, A. (2002). Beyond therapy: Music, spirituality, and health in human experience: A review of literature. *Journal of Music Therapy, 39*(3), 209–240.

Longfield, V. (1995). *The effects of music therapy on pain and mood in hospice patients.* Unpublished master's thesis, St. Louis University, St. Louis, MO.

MacLeod, R. (2008). Setting the context: What do we mean by psychosocial care in palliative care? In M. Lloyd-Williams (Ed.), *Psychosocial issues in palliative care* (2nd ed.). New York: Oxford University Press.

Magill, L. (2001). The use of music therapy to address the suffering in advanced cancer pain. *Journal of Palliative Care, 17*(3), 167–172.

Mandel, S. (1993). The role of the music therapist on the hospice/palliative care team. *Journal of Palliative Care, 9*(4), 37–39.

McNurlen, B. C. (1989). Relationship between the team approach and stress management among hospice workers. *Dissertation Abstracts International, 49*, 9-A.

Moore, R., Staum, M., & Brotons, M. (1992). Music preferences of the elderly: Repertoire, vocal ranges, tempos, and accompaniments for singing. *Journal of Music Therapy, 29*, 236–252.

Munro, S. (1984). *Music therapy in palliative/hospice care.* St. Louis, MO: MMB Music.

Nelson, J. P. (2006). Being in tune with life: Complementary therapy use and well-being in residential hospice residents. *Journal of Holistic Nursing, 24*(3), 152–161.

Nerken, I. R. (1993). Grief and the reflective self: Toward a clearer model of loss resolution and growth. *Death Studies, 17*, 1–26.

Nguyen, J. T. (2003). *The effect of music therapy on end-of-life patients' quality of life, emotional state, and family satisfaction as measured by self report.* Unpublished master's thesis, The Florida State University, Tallahassee.

O'Callaghan, C. (1996). Lyrical themes in songs written by palliative care patients. *Journal of Music Therapy, 33*, 74–92.

O'Callaghan, C. (1997). Therapeutic opportunities associated with the music when using song writing in palliative care. *Music Therapy Perspectives, 15,* 32–38.

O'Callaghan, C. (2009). Objectivist and constructivist music therapy research in oncology and palliative care: An overview and reflection. *Music and Medicine, 1*(1), 41–60.

Okamoto, M. (2004). *The effects of music therapy interventions on grief and spirituality of family members of patients in a hospice setting.* Unpublished master's thesis, Florida State University, Tallahassee.

Parker-Oliver, D., Bronstein, L., & Kurzejeski, L. (2005). Examining variables related to successful collaboration on the hospice team. *Health and Social Work, 30*(4), 278– 291.

Porchet-Munro, S. (1993). Music therapy perspectives in palliative care education. *Journal of Palliative Care, 9*(4), 39–42.

Rando, T. A. (1984). *Grief, dying and death: Clinical interventions for caregivers.* Champaign, IL: Research Press.

Ransford, H. E., & Smith, M. L. (1991). Grief resolution among the bereaved in hospice and hospital wards. *Social Science in Medicine, 32*(3), 295–304.

Ryan, K. L. (1996). *Developing an approach to the use of music therapy with hospice patients in the final phase of life: An examination of how hospice patients from three religious traditions use music and respond to music therapy.* Unpublished master's thesis, Case Western Reserve University, Cleveland, OH.

Salmon, D. (2001). Music therapy as psychospiritual process in palliative care. *Journal of Palliative Care, 17*(3), 142–146.

Salmon, D. (2002, July). *Death and the music therapist: Coping with ongoing loss and suffering.* Paper presented at the meeting of the 10th World Congress of Music Therapy, Oxford, England.

Silverman, M. J. (2009). The use of lyric analysis interventions in contemporary psychiatric music therapy: Descriptive results of songs and objectives for clinical practice. *Music Therapy Perspectives, 27*(1), 55–61.

Smith, M. L. (1984). *The impact of the setting for dying on grief resolution: Hospice versus traditional hospital.* Unpublished doctoral dissertation, University of Southern California.

Speck, P. (2006). Team or group—Spot the difference. In P. Speck (Ed.), *Teamwork in palliative care: Fulfilling or frustrating?* New York: Oxford University Press.

Standley, J., & Jones, J. (2007). *Music techniques in therapy, counseling, and special education.* (3rd ed.). Silver Spring, MD: American Music Therapy Association.

Steinhauser, K. (2002). Initial assessment of a new instrument to measure quality of life at the end of life. *Journal of Palliative Medicine, 5*(6), 829–841.

Thompson, S. (2009). Themes and metaphors in songwriting with clients participating in a psychiatric rehabilitation program. *Music Therapy Perspectives, 27*(1), 4–10.

West, T. M. (1994). Psychological issues in hospice music therapy. *Music Therapy Perspectives, 12,* 117–124.

Wexler, M. M. D. (1989). The use of song in grief therapy with Cibecue White Mountain Apaches. *Music Therapy Perspectives, 7*, 63–66.

Whitall, J. (1991). Songs in palliative care: A spouse's last gift. In K. Bruscia (Ed.), *Case studies in music therapy* (pp. 603–610). Phoenixville, PA: Barcelona.

Wittenberg-Lyles, E., Oliver, D., Demiris, G., & Courtney, K. (2007). Assessing the nature and process of hospice interdisciplinary team meetings. *Journal of Hospice and Palliative Nursing, 9*(1), 17–21.

Wlodarczyk, N. (2007). The effect of music therapy on the spirituality of persons in an in-patient hospice unit as measured by self-report. *Journal of Music Therapy, 44*, 113–122.

Wlodarczyk, N. (2008). *The effect of a live music interaction on the stress levels of hospice staff workers during a hospice interdisciplinary team meeting.* Unpublished manuscript.

Wlodarczyk, N. (2009). The use of music and poetry in life review with hospice patients. *Journal of Poetry Therapy, 22*(3), 133–139.

Wlodarczyk, N. (2010). *The effect of a single-session music therapy group intervention for grief resolution on the disenfranchised grief of hospice workers.* Unpublished doctoral dissertation, The Florida State University, Tallahassee.

Worden, J. W. (2009). *Grief counseling and grief therapy: A handbook for the mental health practitioner* (4th ed.). New York: Springer.

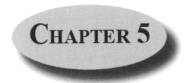

CHAPTER 5

REVIEW OF THE RESEARCH LITERATURE ON PALLIATIVE CARE AND MUSIC THERAPY

This song is the best gift I could have gotten this year. When I hear it, I can picture my husband as if he were right here with me.

—Mrs. R. (wife of hospice patient)

When you play that song, I close my eyes and picture what heaven must look like where there is no pain. —Mrs. J.

Complementary therapies—such as massage therapy, Reiki, art therapy, poetry therapy, aromatherapy, and music therapy—are becoming more common in the hospice setting as interventions to supplement and enhance patient care (Demmer & Sauer, 2002; Mazza, 2001; Nelson, 2006; Tilden, Drach, & Tolle, 2004; Weishaar, 1999). One study revealed that hospice patients and families who received complementary therapies reported a higher satisfaction with overall hospice services (Demmer & Sauer, 2002). Another study suggested that the benefit to the patient comes from the presence of a relationship with the therapist and not necessarily from the responses to the individual complementary therapies themselves (Nelson, 2006). Art therapy, poetry therapy, and music therapy possess a shared component that is vital to the hospice journey: a forum for self-expression. Though all three of these complementary therapies have documented success, to date, music therapy has the largest body of research supporting its efficacy in treating the multidimensional needs of hospice patients (Hilliard, 2001b, 2005; O'Callaghan, 2009).

MUSIC AND QUALITY OF LIFE

Since achieving and maintaining the highest possible quality of life for each patient is the fundamental goal of hospice care, music therapists work to meet this goal in all interventions (Abbott, 1995; Cohen, 2001). *Quality of life* is a comprehensive term that encompasses the wide range of patients' needs: physical, emotional, and spiritual (Byock, 1998; Efficace & Marrone, 2002). Each intervention used with hospice patients is designed to meet both a primary goal, such as increased socialization or decreased perception of pain, and the secondary goal of improved quality of life. Most individuals would agree that enjoying music of their choice on a regular basis improves their quality of life. Similarly, hospice patients may also experience an improved quality of life from routine listening of preferred music recordings.

However, research has shown significant improvements in patients' quality of life as a result of the unique personal interaction with a music therapist who can match live music activities to the patient's changing needs (Hilliard, 2003, 2005). Additionally, live music has been found to be more effective than recorded music in meeting patients' goals (Lee, 2005; Segall, 2007; Standley, 2000).

Quality of life is a complex and multidimensional construct; thus, designing music therapy studies to accurately capture possible effects can be challenging. Furthermore, biased or inadequate sample sizes or inappropriate assessment tools can be confounding variables for research in this area (Field, Clark, Corner, & Davis, 2001). Abbott (1995) found no significant differences on quality of life measures between music therapy recipients and a control group, a total of 28 hospice patients. The researcher concluded that the small sample size may have been a confounding factor, as well as the lengthy questionnaire that seemed to fatigue paticipants. Nguyen (2003) found no significant differences on quality-of-life measures between music therapy and control groups with a total sample size of 20 hospice participants. However, Okamoto (2004) found a significant difference on measures of quality of life in favor of the music therapy group, with a total sample size of 60 participants. The sample size in each of these studies was most likely a factor in their success rate.

In order to evaluate the effects of music therapy on quality of life, length of life in hospice care, and time of death in relation to last music therapy visit, Hilliard (2003) conducted a randomized controlled study with a total of 80 hospice patients. Participants were randomly assigned to a group receiving routine music therapy visits or to a wait-listed control group. Participants in both groups continued to receive all other routine hospice services during the experimental period. All participants completed the Hospice Quality of Life Index–Revised. The functional status of each participant was measured by his or her nurse using the Palliative Performance Scale. Results showed that quality of life was higher for participants receiving music therapy and that these patients' quality of life scores increased over time as they had more music therapy sessions. Participants in the control group experienced a lower quality of life and their quality of life also decreased over time. There were no significant differences between groups on measures of length of life, functional status, or time of death in relation to last music therapy visit.

Another study (Hilliard, 2004b) utilized an ex post facto design to evaluate music therapy recipients' length of life in the hospice program, time of death in relation to last music therapy or social worker visit, and the amount of time the music therapist, as compared to social workers, spent with each participant. Eighty medical records of hospice patients that resided in nursing homes were randomly selected for this study; specifically, 40 records were of patients who had received music therapy, and 40 records were of patients who had not received music therapy. The analysis revealed no significant differences between groups for time of death in relation to last music therapy or social worker visit, but there was a significant difference in length of life in favor of music therapy recipients. Additionally, participants received significantly more music therapy sessions than social work sessions, and music therapists spent more time in direct contact with participants than did social workers.

MUSIC AND LIFE REVIEW

Research has shown that patients usually prefer music that was popular during their early adult years (Gibbons, 1977; Moore, Staum, & Brotons, 1992; Prickett & Bridges, 2000; VanWeelden & Cevasco,

2007). The referential meaning that individuals associate with their preferred music makes it an effective tool for reminiscence, or, as it is commonly referred to in hospice work, life review. The end of one's life is an obvious time for reflection. Hospice patients often enjoy reliving fond memories such as stories about their childhood, how they met their partner, and raising children or grandchildren. They also struggle with unresolved conflicts, estranged relationships, spiritual distress, and fear of how they will be remembered after they are gone (Byock, 2004).

One aspect of music therapy that allows the patient to be in control of the direction of the session is song choice (Hilliard, 2005; Walker & Adamek, 2008). One study reported nine major themes in the song choices by hospice patients and their families: hope, pleasure, the world, reminiscence, relationships, needs and desires, feelings, loss and death, and peace (Bailey, 1984). Familiar music can stimulate discussion of life events and allow the music therapist to guide patients in working through unresolved issues (Abbott, 1995; Walker & Adamek, 2008; Wylie, 1990). Music-assisted life review can also lead to secondary benefits for patients, such as decreased depressive symptoms and decreased feelings of isolation (Ashida, 2000; Clements-Cortés, 2004).

As memories are elicited through familiar music, the music therapist can compile them for use in a songwriting activity. Songwriting can be a useful framework in which to organize and preserve a patient's life story, messages to loved ones, and hopes for future generations (O'Callaghan, 1996; O'Kelly, 2002; Whitall, 1991). Songs written about patients can serve as a way for the whole family to celebrate the patient's life. In a study of hospitalized end-of-life patients, Nguyen (2003) engaged patients in music therapy for life review, wrote an individualized song about each patient and family in their preferred style, and then performed the song at an "end of life celebration" for each patient and family. Measures of participants' perceived quality of life, emotional state, and family satisfaction with music therapy services were compared with those of a no-contact control group. Though there were no significant differences between groups on measure of quality of life, the experimental group had significantly lower anxiety levels and family members reported a 97% satisfaction rate with music therapy services (Nguyen, 2003).

Many hospice patients already engage in some form of journaling or poetry writing as an outlet for expressing feelings about the dying process (Pennebaker, 1997). The music therapist can enhance these practices by setting a patient's words to music. Often "stream of consciousness" writing provides the foundation for a patient-written song. Other times interview-style is a more sucessful approach. The music therapist will use the songwriting method that is most appropriate for each patient's individual needs and ability level. Studies with hospice patients and songwriting have revealed consistent themes in the patient-written lyrics. O'Callaghan (1996) found eight recurring themes in 64 patient-written songs: self-reflections, compliments to others, memories, reflections upon significant others and pets, self-expression of adversity, imagery, and prayers.

Those who are facing the end of life often leave behind adult children and grandchildren and wish to leave advice for them for the future (Byock, 2004). In other cases, hospice patients may still be young adults who desire to leave wishes and life advice for their young children to receive when they are older. In either situation, these sentiments can be expressed in an "ethical will," which is a written statement of a patient's beliefs, values, and hopes for the future for his or her loved ones or community (Baines, 2002). This concept can be combined with music therapy as the music therapist can guide the patient in writing an ethical will, set it to music, and record it for the family to preserve for future generations. Songs of this type may also serve as a healing tool for grieving families after the patient has died (Wlodarczyk, 2009).

Another intervention involving life review and music therapy is the creation of "Living Legacy Projects" (Big Bend Hospice, 2007). These multimedia projects may include recordings of patient-written songs for individual family members, printed song lyrics, photographs, video of patients and families singing together, clips from home movies, artwork, scrapbooking, written or spoken stories, quilting, or any other medium that patients choose to express themselves. The process of creating these projects can provide the patient with a sense of accomplishment, a sense of control regarding how he or she will be remembered by others, and a way to leave lasting memories for loved ones. Living Legacy Projects can also assist patients and family members in saying goodbye.

MUSIC AND PSYCHOSOCIAL ISSUES

Though more commonly used to describe the experiences of the bereaved, Kübler-Ross's (1969) Five Stages of Grief were originally meant to describe the experiences of end-of-life patients. Contrary to a common misconception, Kübler-Ross's stages (denial, anger, bargaining, depression, and acceptance) are not meant to be experienced in a particular order; an individual may skip or repeat any stage throughout the dying process (Bright, 1986; Kübler-Ross, 1969; Worden, 2009). Hospice clinicians typically use the term *anticipatory grief* to describe the gamut of emotions that patients experience as they anticipate death (Hilliard, 2001, 2005; Walker & Adamek, 2008). Patients will have different needs and emotional responses depending on their personal situation, but the need for closure is fairly consistent among hospice patients (Hilliard, 2005). Byock (2004) wrote that there are four phrases that hospice patients and their families should say to each other to promote healing and closure at the end of life: "Please forgive me," "I forgive you," "Thank you," and "I love you." Music therapists can assist patients in expressing these sentiments and achieving a sense of closure through interventions such as music-assisted life review, song choice, songwriting, lyric analysis, and the creation of "Living Legacy Projects" (Abbott, 1995; Ashida, 2000; Bailey, 1984; Big Bend Hospice, 2007; Clements-Cortés, 2004; Nguyen, 2003; O'Callaghan, 1996, 1997; O'Kelly, 2002; Walker & Adamek, 2008; Whitall, 1991; Wlodarczyk, 2009; Wylie, 1990). The hospice music therapy literature is rich in descriptive analyses and case studies describing successful interventions for psychosocial issues. To date, there remains a dearth in quantitative studies testing psychosocial music therapy interventions in this setting.

MUSIC AND SPIRITUALITY

Spirituality has been gaining increased attention in all areas of healthcare, but because of the age-old questions pairing death and spiritual issues, it is especially pertinent to hospice care. Recent studies have shown a general positive correlation between patients' spiritual well-being and physical health outcomes (Anandarajah & Hight, 2001; Edwards & Hall, 2002; Peterman & Fitchett, 2002). Although case studies examining the spiritual aspects of palliative care are quite abundant, there is a deficit in quantitative research on this topic (Wlodarczyk, 2007). As the medical community moves toward a more holistic approach to healthcare—or treatment of the "whole person"—there is expected to be more research on the effect of spirituality on physical health outcomes.

An integral relationship between music and spirituality dates back to the beginning of history (Gilbert, 1977). Music is a natural human expression of emotion and of things for which words are not adequate. It can serve as a symbolic or spiritual language (Salmon, 1993). Music can provide an outlet in which patients can express their spirituality, draw closer to their higher power, and derive feelings of comfort, reassurance, and faith. Hospice patients frequently make associations between music and spirituality (West, 1994). Foxglove and Tyas (2000) wrote that music is "a metaphor for wholeness, symbolizing restoration, transcendence, and relationship."

In an effort to understand the intersection of music, spirituality, and healthcare, Lipe (2002) conducted a comprehensive literature review of 52 articles published between 1973 and 2000. Findings indicated that caregivers view music as a way to support a patient's spiritual needs and to assist them in moving toward spiritual healing. Still, there is limited research regarding the ways that the musical and spiritual aspects of the human experience work together to influence overall patient health (Lipe, 2002). O'Callaghan's (1996) study of songwriting with hospice patients revealed eight lyrical themes from 64 patient-written songs. One of the recurring themes was prayer, specifically "gratitude to God." Results of this study suggest that songwriting is an effective technique for meeting the psychosocial and spiritual needs of hospice patients.

Due to the frequency of requests for spiritual music in hospice music therapy sessions, Wlodarczyk (2007) sought to determine if typical music therapy sessions had a positive impact on hospice patients' sense of spiritual well-being. Participants ($N = 10$), who were hospice inpatients at a 12-bed hospice facility, were used as their own control and responded to a religiously non-specific spiritual well-being questionnaire at the end of four consecutive sessions alternating music and no music. Results of this study showed a statistically significant increase in spiritual well-being scores on music days. In addition, patients initiated spiritual discussion more frequently on music days than on non-music days (Wlodarczyk, 2007).

Given that hospice music therapists work with the entire family in addition to the patient, Okamoto (2004) investigated the effects of music therapy on feelings of grief and spirituality in family members of hospice patients. Participants ($N = 60$) in this study were family members or significant others of hospice patients and were divided into experimental (receiving music therapy services) and control (not receiving music therapy services) groups. A posttest only self-report questionnaire was used to test for differences between the two groups on measures of grief, coping skills, spirituality, satisfaction with hospice care, and perception of the hospice patient's quality of life. Results showed a significant difference between groups for perception of quality of life with the music therapy group being perceived as better than those not receiving music therapy services (Okamoto, 2004).

When dealing with spirituality in hospice care, the music therapist should avoid making assumptions about the patient's beliefs. Though patients may share that they are a member of a particular religious group, it does not automatically imply that they subscribe to all aspects of that specific doctrine (Emblen & Pesut, 2001). In a survey of 310 congregation members representing three churches of differing denominations, results suggested that church attendance does not indicate the desired level of spiritual support of an individual. Additionally, those who felt that they were receiving spiritual support listed unique sources above and beyond those provided through church attendance (Fiala, 2002).

Music therapy can be used for spiritual support in the hospice setting by providing an opportunity for worship. Hospice patients quickly become too ill to attend spiritual services or participate in church events that may have been an important aspect of their lives prior to their diagnosis. Isolation from one's spiritual community can lead to spiritual distress, loneliness, and depression (Wlodarczyk, 2007). Music therapy sessions can allow patients to participate in their favorite spiritual music and simultaneously increase their spiritual well-being and their level of socialization. Music therapists must master a wide range of spiritual repertoire in order to adequately meet patients' needs. Though the majority of patients seen tend to request spiritual music from Christian denominations, it is important to learn songs from other traditions as well (Ryan, 1996).

A music therapy session with a hospice patient often involves a time of music and prayer. The patient may be moved to meditate or pray silently or aloud during the music. Oftentimes a patient has a desire to pray but may find it an uncomfortable or unfamiliar thing to do. Music can create a safe environment in which patients feel comfortable to express their spirituality in whatever manner they choose. Salmon (2001) wrote of the importance of creating a "sacred space" with music in which patients may safely explore their spiritual awareness. Music can also be a catalyst for emotional catharsis during spiritual exploration. Music therapists can structure a session to uncover and work though any issues of spiritual distress that the patient may be feeling. Music can also assist patients in reminiscence of spiritual events throughout their lifetime, such as baptisms, confirmations, and even weddings and funerals. The bedside vigil when a patient is imminently dying is another deeply spiritual time of the hospice journey (Krout, 2003). At this time the music therapist may facilitate the soft singing of hymns or provide soothing background music while family members pray or speak words of love to the patient. The music therapist should be positioned in a far corner of the room so that the focus of this session is the interaction between the patient and family members, with the music therapist providing only the structure and the facilitation.

MUSIC FOR PAIN AND SYMPTOM MANAGEMENT

Pain and symptom management is a primary goal in hospice care and an important component to maintaining high quality of life for patients and their families. Though hospice patients represent a variety of terminal diagnoses, pain control—for either acute or chronic pain—is usually a goal at some point for each patient. Hospice nurses are considered to be experts in pain control and work diligently to ensure that each hospice patient's life is as pain-free as possible. Each member of the IDT is responsible for assessing, documenting, and reporting a patient's pain level at each visit (Groen, 2007). Other physiological symptoms that are commonly seen in hospice patients include anxiety, agitation, nausea and vomiting, and shortness of breath (Hilliard, 2005; Magill, 2001; Walker & Adamek, 2008).

Music is most effective for pain management when a patient experiences pain that is mild to moderate and is less effective for severe pain (Standley, 2000). Music therapists use music for pain management (Walker & Adamek, 2008)

- as a stimulus for focus of attention or distraction
- to facilitate relaxation
- as a masking agent
- as a positive environmental stimulus

A common music therapy intervention for pain and symptom management is the use of the Iso-Principle, which involves matching the tempo (speed) and volume (intensity) of the music to the patient's current level of symptom intensity and then gradually altering the music to bring the patient to the desired physiological state (Davis, Gfeller, & Thaut, 2008). Similar to other music therapy interventions, the Iso-Principle is most effective when using patient-preferred music (Standley, 2000). Other music therapy interventions used for pain and symptom management include music as distraction, music-assisted progressive music relaxation (PMR), and music paired with guided imagery for relaxation.

Many descriptive articles and case studies have outlined the use of music therapy for pain and symptom management in hospice patients (Groen, 2007; Hilliard, 2001b; Magill, 2001; Michel & Chesky, 1995; O'Callaghan, 1996; Starr, 1999; Trauger-Querry & Haghighi, 1999; Wylie & Blum, 1986), but minimal quantitative studies have investigated these practices. Longfield (1995) compared listening to recorded music versus no music for pain management in eight hospice patients who served as their own control. Results showed a significant difference between conditions, with dependent measures of pain, fatigue, anxiety, and energy improving on music days. Lee (2005), in a study of 40 hospice patients, found that live music therapy utilizing the Iso-Principle was significantly more effective than recorded music in reducing pain and anxiety. Batzner (2003) studied the effect of therapist vocal improvisation on the discomfort behaviors of hospice patients and found that vocal improvisation with live guitar accompaniment decreased discomfort behaviors as indicated by graphic analysis. Calovini (1993) examined the effect of a single music therapy session on the anxiety of hospice patients ($N = 11$) and found no significant differences, citing that single music therapy sessions were limited in their ability to effect change in chronic symptoms. Conversely, Krout (2001) found a significant reduction for measures of pain and anxiety in single music therapy sessions with 80 hospice patients, suggesting that an adequate sample size may produce more accurate results.

To evaluate the effects of music on pain relief and relaxation, Curtis (1986) conducted a study in which 9 terminally ill patients were subjected to three conditions: control (no intervention), a recording of ambient hospital sounds, and calm, preferred instrumental music. Each participant received all conditions and was randomly assigned to one of two condition orders. Participants completed self-report measures of pain relief, physical comfort, contentment, and relaxation. Results of the statistical analysis indicated no significant differences between treatment variables, but a graphical analysis of individual responses indicated that the music condition was most preferred. Another quantitative study (Horne-Thompson & Grocke, 2008) used a randomized controlled design to examine the effect of music therapy on anxiety in patients ($N = 25$) who were terminally ill. Results demonstrated a significant difference between groups in favor of the music therapy condition for self-report measures of anxiety, pain, tiredness, and drowsiness, but no significant difference between groups for the physiological measure of heart rate.

In a landmark quantitative study utilizing a computerized database program and standardized data collection forms, Gallagher, Lagman, Walsh, Davis, and LeGrand (2006) assessed the effects of music therapy with hospice patients ($N = 200$) on a variety of dependent variables. Results of the analysis showed that music therapy significantly improved anxiety, body movement, facial expression, mood, pain, shortness of breath, and verbalizations. Sessions with participants' family members were also evaluated and music therapy significantly improved family members' facial expressions, mood, and verbalizations. This study supports the use of large sample sizes and a computerized database to enhance hospice music therapy research.

Two different studies investigated the effects of music on non-responsive or comatose hospice patients. Kerr (2004) compared two different conditions—silence versus recorded music chosen by the researcher—on 10 non-responsive hospice patients. Results showed significantly lowered physiological measures of heart rate and respiration rate under the music condition. Segall (2007) compared the effects of silence, patient-preferred recorded music, and patient-preferred live music on 10 non-responsive hospice patients. Results showed no significant differences between the three conditions for measures of heart rate or respiration rate. However, the preferred live music condition was significantly more effective than both the preferred recorded music condition and the baseline condition in eliciting patients' most alert states as measured by a behavioral observation coding system. Both of these studies support the continued use of music therapy with hospice patients who become non-responsive (Kerr, 2004; Segall, 2007).

MUSIC AND BEREAVEMENT

Music and other art forms—often referred to as "the healing arts"—are commonly integrated into grief counseling, grief therapy, and grief support groups (Bertman, 1999; Bolton, 2008; Grebin & Vogel, 2006/2007; Rogers, 2007). Music therapy is an intervention that is well suited to assist mourners in working through the pain of grief due to its many modes for expression of grief feelings and its ability to provide a positive connection to the deceased (Bright, 1986; Curtis, 1989; Hilliard, 2005; Lochner & Stevenson, 1988; Loyst, 1989; Mandel, 1993; Rogers, 2007; Smeijsters & van den Hurk, 1999). Since music has always been a natural part of bereavement rituals (Aborampah, 1999; Amir, 1998; Berger, 2006; Jones, Baker, & Day, 2004), it is a logical progression for music therapists to be involved in the field of grief counseling (Berger, 2006). Music therapy in grief counseling employs the use of client-preferred music, which may include songs from memorial services, favorite songs of the deceased, or songs that were created or improvised during music therapy sessions with the deceased (Bright, 1999, 2002; Krout, 2005). Each music therapy intervention can be tailored to suit the client's age, music preference, and specific type of loss (Berger, 2006; Bright, 1999).

Participation in music therapy groups has been effective in reducing grief reactions for children who have experienced the loss of a loved one (Burke, 1991; Loewy, 2004). Research has suggested that a music-based curriculum addressing death education, mood, and behaviors of grieving children may lower grief symptoms and significantly improve problem behaviors in the home (Hilliard, 2001a). Studies utilizing an Orff-Schulwerk approach to music therapy groups for grieving children have shown positive effects, such as consistent group attendance, on-task behavior, and a reduction of grief symptoms (Hilliard, 2007; Register & Hilliard, 2008). Musical games and improvisation have also been effective with grieving children, including bereaved siblings (Mayhew, 2005).

Music therapy has demonstrated efficacy in addressing the grief symptoms of adolescents as well (Dalton & Krout, 2005; Shaller & Smith, 2002; Skewes, 2001). Primary needs of grieving adolescents include emotional expression, development of effective coping mechanisms, and development of supportive peer relationships (Shaller & Smith, 2002). Music is a successful tool with adolescents because it is naturally reinforcing, inherently promotes self-expression, and strengthens the bonds of peer relationships in a group setting. For these reasons, structured music therapy sessions are able to facilitate meeting primary needs of grieving adolescents (Shaller & Smith, 2002). Appropriate music therapy interventions for this age group include structured drumming, instrument improvisation, songwriting, and lyric analysis (Dalton & Krout, 2005; Shaller & Smith, 2002; Skewes, 2001).

An investigation by Skewes (2001) explored group improvisation and group music sharing in music therapy sessions with 6 bereaved adolescents over the course of 10 weeks. Following participation in the group, the researcher conducted in-depth interviews with the participants that were then transcribed and analyzed for thematic content. The analysis revealed that participants were able to express and effectively deal with their grief feelings because the group met their developmentally appropriate needs for fun, freedom, control, and group cohesion. Participants also shared that the ability to share grief feelings through music without relying on words was helpful in achieving grief resolution and also in strengthening continued bonds with their loved ones who had died.

It is often difficult to find appropriate measures for music therapy studies. Dalton and Krout (2005) designed and piloted a music therapy-focused grief processing assessment instrument for bereaved adolescents who received group songwriting as an intervention for grief symptoms. The resultant instrument, the Grief Process Scale (GPS), has shown promise as a tool for the evaluation of the effectiveness of music therapy interventions with adolescent groups in future research studies. Development of the scale was derived from analysis of 123 songs written by bereaved adolescents during music therapy sessions. Thirty self-statements were generated from the song analysis, which corresponded to five grief process content areas taken from the grief literature. Statements on the GPS were then organized into these content areas. A continuous line marked from 0 to 100 connects the identifiers "easy" and "hard" at either end of each statement. Participants mark the line in response to statements such as "Since my loved one died, letting myself cry and feel my sadness about the death is . . ." The GPS can be used as a pretest and posttest to evaluate the effectiveness of music therapy treatment with bereaved adolescents (Dalton & Krout, 2005).

Music therapy sessions with grieving adults can take place in either a group setting or one-on-one (Bright, 1986, 2002; Hanser, 1990; Mandel, 1993; McDonnell, 1984). In a group setting, music can create powerful change through interpersonal interaction, bonding, empathy, and emotional expression (Grebin & Vogel, 2006/2007). Music therapist-composed original songs have been used to create participant connections, explore session topics, and help facilitate group rituals in adult bereavement groups (Krout, 2005). Vocal and instrumental improvisation has been used to assist individual adult clients in communicating previously suppressed feelings and establishing a new personal identity after the death of a loved one (Smeijsters & van den Hurk, 1999).

Since the grief literature points to participation in ritual as an important step toward grief resolution (Castle & Phillips, 2003), music therapists working with the bereaved can incorporate ritual elements into music therapy sessions. In the instance of an ongoing group, a grief ritual could be planned for the final group meeting as a way to commemorate loved ones who have died and also the bonds and time that were shared by the group participants. Krout (2005) described several rituals used in his work with bereaved adolescents and adults, including creating a pathway lined by stones on which participants have written the names of deceased loved ones, writing messages to participants' loved ones on biodegradable paper boats and floating them on an available body of water, and creating a group product that was observable to others on the beach. Live music facilitated by the music therapist, such as singing or group drumming, combined with these rituals can be a powerful vehicle for healing and group transformation.

Songwriting has been a popular and successful music therapy intervention for bereaved persons across age groups and is a common practice in grief support groups led by music therapists. Songs may be pre-composed for a group by the music therapist with a specific goal or topic in mind (Krout, 2005), written as an activity with a single client (Smeijsters & van den Hurk, 1999), or created as a group process during a music therapy group session (Bright, 1999; Dalton & Krout, 2005, 2006). O'Callaghan (2008) examined the similarities present in lullabies and laments composed during music therapy sessions with grieving adults. The researcher coined the term *lullament* to describe the interconnected qualities of both song types as they pertain to grief expressions in client-composed songs. Songwriting can be used to communicate a final goodbye to loved ones, thus aiding the bereaved in working through the pain of grief (O'Callaghan, 2008; Whitall, 1991), which is the first task of mourning (Worden, 2009).

Dalton and Krout (2006) outlined and developed a specific grief songwriting protocol to be used with bereaved adolescents. Their project involved three phases: a descriptive thematic analysis of 123 songs written by bereaved adolescents, comparison of thematic material from these songs with existing grief models, and the subsequent development of the Grief Song-Writing Process Protocol (GSWP) based upon these findings. The adolescents involved in this study received weekly music therapy and grief counseling over the course of 36 months. The actual songwriting process involved participants making decisions about the creation of lyrics and the type of music to be used. They were instructed to use the song lyrics to express their concerns regarding the death of their loved one and how they were coping with the death. The researchers organized themes from the participant-written lyrics into five content areas taken from the grief literature: understanding, feeling, remembering, integrating, and growing. The GSWP was developed from these outcomes and involved devoting a music therapy session to each of the five content areas by writing a song based on that theme and discussing both the process and the product (Dalton & Krout, 2006).

MUSIC THERAPY FOR HOSPICE WORKERS

Music therapy has been shown to be effective with hospice patients and families, but it is also beginning to be explored as an intervention for hospice staff as well. Workplace wellness programs have generally been associated with cost-savings and decreased employee absenteeism (Aldana, Merrill, Price, Hardy, & Hager, 2005). Music and music-assisted relaxation techniques have been shown to significantly decrease arousal due to stress (Pelletier, 2004), and music therapy has also been shown to reduce stress and anxiety in a variety of individuals and settings (Kim, 2006; Robb, 2000). These conclusions provide support for the exploration of music therapy as an intervention for stress, burnout, and compassion fatigue in hospice workers (Hilliard, 2006).

Since music-assisted relaxation has been effective in patients, Palmer (2003) investigated the effect of music listening paired with taped guided relaxation in a pilot study with hospice workers. Participation took place at the hospice building during participants' lunch hour. Participants ($N = 21$) were seated in padded chairs in a dimly lit room during the intervention. The type of music that was used during the guided relaxation was either classical or New Age music and was chosen by the researcher. Pretest and posttest measures of mood and global stress were taken as well as answers to open-ended questions. Results showed a significant reduction on dependent measures of mood, affect, and global stress for participants from pretest to posttest. Though participants did not necessarily prefer the music that was used for the intervention, they still found the experience to be generally relaxing.

Many hospice music therapists regularly incorporate some type of live music at staff meetings, though to date no studies were found that attempted to quantify possible effects. Wlodarczyk (2008) studied the effect of live music at the beginning of hospice IDT meetings on the self-reported stress levels of hospice workers. This study used a complete reversal design over the course of four consecutive weekly meetings. Participants ($N = 23$) indicated their current level of stress on a visual analogue scale at the start of each meeting. Results of self-reported stress levels showed no significant difference between experimental and control conditions; however, free responses collected from participants were 100% positive in favor of the music. Results of this study do not support live music in IDT meetings as an intervention for stress reduction, but do support the practice as one that is enjoyed by hospice workers and therefore should continue to be offered. Future studies on this particular practice could clarify if the music may be improving mood or morale versus stress for hospice workers.

Following the support group model that is commonly used with hospice families, Hilliard (2006) looked at the effects of group music therapy on compassion fatigue and team building in one sample of hospice workers. Participants in this study ($N = 17$) were nurses, social workers, and chaplains who had been employed at the hospice for more than 1 year. Due to the distance between the two hospice offices, randomization to groups was not possible for this study. Instead, each office was assigned to one of two experimental conditions and participants attended the group that was provided at their home office. One group received improvisational music therapy sessions and the other group received structured or didactic music therapy sessions. Sessions were provided weekly for 6 weeks. There were no significant differences on dependent measures between the two different experimental groups. There was also no significant difference in compassion fatigue for each individual group from pretest to posttest. However, there was a significant improvement in team building for both experimental groups from pretest to posttest (Hilliard, 2006).

Music therapy has also been preliminarily explored as an intervention for the buildup of unresolved grief in hospice workers. Wlodarczyk (2010) tested the effect of a single-session music therapy group on hospice workers' feelings of grief resolution, burnout, compassion fatigue, and perception of work environment. Participants ($N = 68$) were members of the IDT and attended either a randomly assigned experimental group ($n = 34$) or a randomly assigned control group ($n = 34$). Results indicated a statistically significant reduction for the grief resolution subscale of "personal sacrifice burden" from pretest to posttest for the experimental group. Results of this study also included a thematic analysis of participant-written song lyrics and messages to patients who had died. This analysis revealed common themes surrounding the meaningfulness of hospice work, which participants indicated outweighed the sadness that is also encountered as part of their jobs.

Research with hospice workers presents some of the same limitations as research with hospice patients and bereaved persons: difficulty establishing randomization, lack of an unbiased sample, and attrition of participants resulting in small sample sizes (Field et al., 2001; Hilliard, 2003; Wlodarczyk, 2008). The nature of hospice work leads to unpredictable schedule changes for employees as they quickly adjust and respond to priority patients' needs. This flexibility in scheduling benefits patient care but makes it difficult for hospice workers to participate in research that requires attendance at multiple sessions. Therefore, it is suggested that researchers with hospice workers attempt to design interventions that can be effective in a single session (Wlodarczyk, 2008, 2010). Also, since research indicates that interventions with hospice workers are most effective when facilitated by a non-staff member, providing groups of this type could be an additional income source for contract music therapists.

CONCLUSION

The overall body of evidence for the continued use of music therapy in hospice and palliative care is strong and will continue to mature. Benefits to both hospice patients and their families are receiving increased attention due to journal publications, conference presentations, and "word of mouth" by those who have seen it work firsthand (Hilliard, 2004a). Often the most effective method of "selling" music therapy is by having patients or family members share their experiences with others. Many hospice music therapy programs have grown from a single music therapist on staff to several additional positions, primarily due to the impact of positive patient and family testimony. Patient and family satisfaction with music therapy can improve the overall impression of the medical facility (Gallagher, Huston, Nelson, Walsh, & Steele, 2001; Nguyen, 2003). Consequently, satisfied music therapy recipients can lead to increased opportunities for donations and other types of fundraising for the continued support of the program.

Research has indicated that there are hospice administrators who would like to add music therapy to their available hospice services but are unsure how to fund the program (Hilliard, 2004a). Music therapists need to become proactive in improving their knowledge and understanding of the business aspects of hospice organizations, methods of reimbursement, and other sources of funding such as acquiring donations and grants. In his text on hospice music therapy, Hilliard (2005) provides a comprehensive guide to music therapy program design and development for hospice settings. Suggestions include conducting a macro-assessment of the agency's needs and available resources, assessing the business structure and tax status, and developing a business plan that fits the profile of the hospice to be solicited (Hilliard, 2005). Knowing the audience is also an important factor in successful business meetings. Hospice social workers may be more impressed by detailed case studies, while physicians will want to see quantitative data that supports effective use of music therapy. Hospice administrators will be interested in any projected cost-savings as a result of adding a music therapy program to their plan of care (Romo & Gifford, 2007).

The role of a hospice music therapist is multifaceted and includes providing direct patient care, educating the hospice team and the community about the benefits of music therapy, developing and maintaining research-based cutting-edge skills, and supporting hospice goals through first-rate documentation practices (Mandel, 1993; O'Callaghan, 2001, 2009). Since hospice care is ubiquitous to healthcare settings, music therapists employed by a hospice have opportunities to visit patients in a variety of environments including hospitals, nursing homes, private homes, group homes, psychological treatment centers, and hospice inpatient facilities. This versatility makes hospice work an attractive choice of vocation for music therapists, but also requires them to have a wide range of skills and repertoire. Many hospice music therapists feel drawn to hospice work as "a calling," and dedication to the hospice mission produces clinicians who are ready and willing to meet the demands of the job (Junkin, 2006).

REFERENCES

Abbott, C. M. (1995). *The effects of music therapy on the perceived quality of life of patients with terminal illness in a hospice setting.* Unpublished master's thesis, Western Michigan University, Kalamazoo.

Aborampah, O. (1999). Women's roles in the mourning rituals of the Akan of Ghana. *Ethnology, 38*(3), 257–271.

Aldana, S. G., Merrill, R. M., Price, K. P., Hardy, A., & Hager, R. (2005). Financial impact of a comprehensive multisite workplace health promotion program. *Preventative Medicine, 40*, 131–137.

Amir, D. (1998). The use of Israeli folksongs in dealing with women's bereavement and loss in music therapy. In D. Dokter (Ed.), *Arts therapies, refugees and migrants: Reaching across borders* (pp. 217–235). London: Jessica Kingsley.

Anandarajah, G., & Hight, E. (2001). Spirituality and medical practice: Using the HOPE questions as a practical tool for spiritual assessment. *American Family Physician, 63*(1), 81–88.

Ashida, S. (2000). The effect of reminiscence music therapy sessions on changes in depressive symptoms in elderly persons with dementia. *Journal of Music Therapy, 37*(3), 170–182.

Bailey, L. M. (1984). The use of songs in music therapy with cancer patients and their families. *Music Therapy, 4*, 5–17.

Baines, B. (2002). *Ethical wills: Putting your values on paper.* Cambridge, MA: Perseus Books Group.

Batzner, K. W. (2003). *The effect of therapist vocal improvisation on discomfort behaviors of in-patient hospice clients.* Unpublished master's thesis, University of Kansas, Lawrence.

Berger, J. S. (2006). *Music of the soul: Composing life out of loss.* New York: Brunner- Routledge.

Bertman, S. L. (Ed.). (1999). *Grief and the healing arts: Creativity as therapy.* Amityville, NY: Baywood.

Big Bend Hospice, Inc. (2007). *Voice of the heart: Legacy guide and journal.* [Brochure]. Tallahassee, FL: Author.

Bolton, G. (Ed.). (2008). *Dying, bereavement, and the healing arts.* London: Jessica Kingsley.

Bright, R. (1986). *Grieving: A handbook for those who care.* St Louis, MO: MMB Music.

Bright, R. (1999). Music therapy in grief resolution. *Bulletin of the Menninger Clinic, 63*(4), 481–498.

Bright, R. (2002). *Supportive eclectic music therapy for grief and loss: A practical handbook for professionals.* St Louis, MO: MMB Music.

Burke, K. (1991). Music therapy in working through a preschooler's grief: Expressing grief and confusion. In K. Bruscia (Ed.), *Case studies in music therapy.* Phoenixville, PA: Barcelona.

Byock, I. (1998). Measuring quality of life for patients with terminal illness: The Missoula-VITAS® Quality of Life Index. *Palliative Medicine, 12*, 231–244.

Byock, I. (2004). *The four things that matter most: A book about living.* New York: Simon & Schuster.

Calovini, B. S. (1993). *The effect of participation in one music therapy session on state anxiety in hospice patients.* Unpublished master's thesis, Case Western Reserve University, Cleveland, OH.

Castle, J., & Phillips, W. L. (2003). Grief rituals: Aspects that facilitate adjustment to bereavement. *Journal of Loss and Trauma, 8*, 41–71.

Clements-Cortés, A. (2004). The use of music in facilitating emotional expression in the terminally ill. *American Journal of Hospice and Palliative Medicine, 21*(4), 255–260.

Cohen, S. (2001). Changes in quality of life following admission to palliative care units. *Palliative Medicine, 15*, 363–371.

Curtis, S. (1989). Music therapy in grief and stress management. In J. Martin (Ed.), *The next step forward: Music therapy with the terminally ill*. Bronx, NY: Calvary Hospital.

Curtis, S. L. (1986). The effect of music on pain relief and relaxation of the terminally ill. *Journal of Music Therapy, 23*, 10–24.

Dalton, T. A., & Krout, R. E. (2005). Development of the Grief Process Scale through music therapy songwriting with bereaved adolescents. *The Arts in Psychotherapy, 32*(2), 131–143.

Dalton, T. A., & Krout, R. E. (2006). The grief song-writing process with bereaved adolescents: An integrated grief model and music therapy protocol. *Music Therapy Perspectives, 24*(2), 94–107.

Davis, W. B., Gfeller, K. E., & Thaut, M. H. (Eds.). (2008). *An introduction to music therapy theory and practice* (3rd ed.). Silver Spring, MD: American Music Therapy Association.

Demmer, C., & Sauer, J. (2002). Assessing complementary therapy services in a hospice program. *American Journal of Hospice and Palliative Medicine, 19*(5), 306–314.

Edwards, K., & Hall, T. (2002). The Spiritual Assessment Inventory: A theistic model and measure for assessing spiritual development. *Journal for the Scientific Study of Religion, 41*(2), 341–357.

Efficace, F., & Marrone, R. (2002). Spiritual issues and quality of life assessment in cancer care. *Death Studies, 26*, 743–756.

Emblen, J., & Pesut, B. (2001). Strengthening transcendent meaning: A model for the spiritual nursing care of patients experiencing suffering. *Journal of Holistic Nursing, 19*(1), 42–56.

Fiala, W. (2002). The Religious Support Scale: Construction, validation and cross-validation. *American Journal of Community Psychology, 30*(6), 761–783.

Field, D., Clark, D., Corner, J., & Davis, C. (Eds.). (2001). *Researching palliative care*. Buckingham, UK: Open University Press.

Foxglove, T., & Tyas, B. (2000). Using music as a spiritual tool in palliative care. *European Journal of Palliative Care, 7*(2), 63–65.

Gallagher, L. M., Huston, M. J., Nelson, K. A., Walsh, D., & Steele, A. (2001). Music therapy in palliative medicine. *Supportive Care in Cancer, 9*(3), 156–161.

Gallagher, L. M., Lagman, R., Walsh, D., Davis, M. P., & LeGrand, S. B. (2006). The clinical effects of music therapy in palliative medicine. *Supportive Care in Cancer, 14*(8), 859–866.

Gibbons, A. C. (1977). Pop music preferences of elderly persons. *Journal of Music Therapy, 14*, 180–189.

Gilbert, J. (1977). Music therapy perspectives on death and dying. *Journal of Music Therapy, 14*(4), 165–171.

Grebin, M., & Vogel, J. E. (2006/2007). Bereavement groups and their benefits: Enhancing connection through creativity. *Journal of Creativity in Mental Health, 2*(1), 61–73.

Groen, K. M. (2007). Pain assessment and management in end of life care: A survey of assessment and treatment practices in hospice music therapy. *Journal of Music Therapy, 44*, 90–112.

Hanser, S. B. (1990). A music therapy strategy for depressed older adults in the community. *Journal of Applied Gerontology, 9*(3), 283–298.

Hilliard, R. E. (2001a). The effects of music therapy-based bereavement groups on mood and behavior of grieving children: A pilot study. *Journal of Music Therapy, 38*, 291–306.

Hilliard, R. E. (2001b). The use of music therapy in meeting the multidimensional needs of hospice patients and families. *Journal of Palliative Care, 17*(3), 161–166.

Hilliard, R. E. (2003). The effects of music therapy on quality of life and length of life of hospice patients diagnosed with terminal cancer. *Journal of Music Therapy, 40*, 113–137.

Hilliard, R. E. (2004a). Hospice administrators' knowledge of music therapy: A comparative analysis of surveys. *Music Therapy Perspectives, 22*(2), 104–108.

Hilliard, R. E. (2004b). A post-hoc analysis of music therapy services for residents in nursing homes receiving hospice care. *Journal of Music Therapy, 41*, 266–281.

Hilliard, R. E. (2005). *Hospice and palliative care music therapy: A guide to program development and clinical care.* Cherry Hill, NJ: Jeffrey Books.

Hilliard, R. E. (2006). The effect of music therapy sessions on compassion fatigue and team building of professional hospice caregivers. *The Arts in Psychotherapy, 33*, 395–401.

Hilliard, R. E. (2007). The effects of Orff-based music therapy and social work groups on childhood grief symptoms and behaviors. *Journal of Music Therapy, 44*(2), 123–138.

Horne-Thompson, A., & Grocke, D. (2008). The effect of music therapy on anxiety in patients who are terminally ill. *Journal of Palliative Medicine, 11*(4), 582–590.

Jones, C., Baker, F., & Day, T. (2004). From healing rituals to music therapy: Bridging the cultural divide between therapist and young Sudanese refugees. *The Arts in Psychotherapy, 31*, 89–100.

Junkin, J. S. (2006). *The impact of a clinician's mourning on music therapy treatment.* Unpublished master's thesis, Drexel University, Philadelphia, PA.

Kerr, S. E. (2004). *The effect of music on non-responsive patients in a hospice setting.* Unpublished master's thesis, The Florida State University, Tallahassee, FL.

Kim, S. A. (2006). *The effect of music listening on mood state and relaxation of hospice patients and caregivers.* Unpublished master's thesis, The Florida State University, Tallahassee, FL.

Krout, R. (2001). The effects of single-session music therapy interventions on the observed and self-reported levels of pain control, physical comfort, and relaxation of hospice patients. *American Journal of Hospice and Palliative Medicine, 18*(6), 383–390.

Krout, R. (2003). Music therapy with imminently dying hospice patients and their families: Facilitating release near the time of death. *American Journal of Hospice and Palliative Medicine, 20*(2), 129–134.

Krout, R. (2005). Applications of music therapist-composed songs in creating participant connections and facilitating goals and rituals during one-time bereavement support groups and programs. *Music Therapy Perspectives, 23*, 118–128.

Kübler-Ross, E. (1969). *On death and dying.* New York: Macmillan.

Lee, H. J. (2005). *The effect of life music via the iso-principle on pain management in palliative care as measured by self report using a graphic rating scale (GRS) and pulse rate.* Unpublished master's thesis, The Florida State University, Tallahassee, FL.

Lipe, A. (2002). Beyond therapy: Music, spirituality, and health in human experience: A review of literature. *Journal of Music Therapy, 39*(3), 209–240.

Lochner, C. W., & Stevenson, R. G. (1988). Music as a bridge to wholeness. *Death Studies, 12*, 173–180.

Loewy, J. (2004). Music therapy to help traumatized children and caregivers. In N. L. Webb's (Ed.), *Mass trauma and violence: Helping families and children cope* (pp. 191–215). New York: Guilford Press.

Longfield, V. (1995). *The effects of music therapy on pain and mood in hospice patients.* Unpublished master's thesis, St. Louis University, St. Louis, MO.

Loyst, D. (1989). A time to remember: Music therapy in bereavement follow-up. In J. Martin (Ed.), *The next step forward: Music therapy with the terminally ill.* Bronx, NY: Calvary Hospital.

Magill, L. (2001). The use of music therapy to address the suffering in advanced cancer pain. *Journal of Palliative Care, 17*(3), 167–172.

Mandel, S. (1993). Music therapy: Variations on a theme. *Journal of Palliative Care, 9*(4), 37–55.

Mayhew, J. (2005). A creative response to loss: Developing a music therapy group for bereaved siblings. In M. Pavlicevic (Ed.), *Music therapy in children's hospices* (pp. 62–80). London: Jessica Kingsley.

Mazza, N. (2001). The place of the poetic in dealing with death and loss. *Journal of Poetry Therapy, 15*(1), 29–35.

McDonnell, L. (1984). Music therapy with trauma patients and their families on a pediatric service. *Music Therapy, 4*, 55–63.

Michel, D. E., & Chesky, K. S. (1995). A survey of music therapists using music for pain relief. *The Arts in Psychotherapy, 22*(1), 49–51.

Moore, R., Staum, M., & Brotons, M. (1992). Music preferences of the elderly: Repertoire, vocal ranges, tempos, and accompaniments for singing. *Journal of Music Therapy, 29*, 236–252.

Nelson, J. P. (2006). Being in tune with life: Complementary therapy use and well-being in residential hospice residents. *Journal of Holistic Nursing, 24*(3), 152–161.

Nguyen, J. T. (2003). *The effect of music therapy on end-of-life patients' quality of life, emotional state, and family satisfaction as measured by self report.* Unpublished master's thesis, The Florida State University, Tallahassee, FL.

O'Callaghan, C. (1996). Lyrical themes in songs written by palliative care patients. *Journal of Music Therapy, 33*, 74–92.

O'Callaghan, C. (1997). Therapeutic opportunities associated with the music when using song writing in palliative care. *Music Therapy Perspectives, 15*, 32–38.

O'Callaghan, C. (2001). Bringing music to life: A study of music therapy and palliative care experiences in a cancer hospital. *Journal of Palliative Care, 17*(3), 155–160.

O'Callaghan, C. (2008). Lullament: Lullaby and lament therapeutic qualities actualized through music therapy. *American Journal of Hospice and Palliative Medicine, 25*(2), 93–99.

O'Callaghan, C. (2009). Objectivist and constructivist music therapy research in oncology and palliative care: An overview and reflection. *Music and Medicine, 1*(1), 41–60.

Okamoto, M. (2004). *The effects of music therapy interventions on grief and spirituality of family members of patients in a hospice setting.* Unpublished master's thesis, The Florida State University, Tallahassee, FL.

O'Kelly, J. (2002). Music therapy in palliative care: Current perspectives. *International Journal of Palliative Nursing, 8*(3), 130–136.

Palmer, J. A. (2003). *Music therapy as a coping mechanism for hospice workers: A pilot study.* Unpublished master's thesis, State University of New York at Buffalo, Buffalo, NY.

Pelletier, C. (2004). The effect of music on decreasing arousal due to stress: A meta-analysis. *Journal of Music Therapy, 41*(3), 192–214.

Pennebaker, J. W. (1997). Writing about emotional experiences as a therapeutic process. *Psychological Science, 8*(3), 162–166.

Peterman, A., & Fitchett, G. (2002). Measuring spiritual well-being in people with cancer: The functional assessment of the chronic illness therapy-spiritual well-being scale (FACIT-Sp). *Annals of Behavioral Medicine, 24*(1), 49–58.

Prickett, C. A., & Bridges, M. S. (2000). Song repertoire across the generations: A comparison of music therapy majors' and senior citizens' recognitions. *Journal of Music Therapy, 37,* 196–204.

Register, D., & Hilliard, R. E. (2008). Using Orff-based techniques in children's bereavement groups: A cognitive-behavioral music therapy approach. *The Arts in Psychotherapy, 35,* 162–170.

Robb, S. L. (2000). Music assisted progressive muscle relaxation, music listening, and silence: A comparison of relaxation techniques. *Journal of Music Therapy, 37*(1), 1–21.

Rogers, E. (Ed.). (2007). *The art of grief: The use of expressive arts in a grief support group.* New York: Routledge.

Romo, R., & Gifford, L. (2007). A cost-benefit analysis of music therapy in a home hospice. *Nursing Economics, 25*(6), 353–358.

Ryan, K. L. (1996). *Developing an approach to the use of music therapy with hospice patients in the final phase of life: An examination of how hospice patients from three religious traditions use music and respond to music therapy.* Unpublished master's thesis, Case Western Reserve University, Cleveland, OH.

Salmon, D. (1993). Music and emotion in palliative care. *Journal of Palliative Care, 9*(4), 48–52.

Salmon, D. (2001). Music therapy as psychospiritual process in palliative care. *Journal of Palliative Care, 17*(3), 142–146.

Segall, L. (2007). *The effect of patient preferred live versus recorded music on non-responsive patients in the hospice setting as evidenced by physiological and behavioural states.* Unpublished master's thesis, The Florida State University, Tallahassee, FL.

Shaller, J., & Smith, C. R. (2002). Music therapy with adolescents experiencing loss. *The Forum: Association for Death Education and Counselling, 28*(5), 1–4.

Skewes, K. (2001). *The experience of group music therapy for six bereaved adolescents.* Unpublished doctoral dissertation, The University of Melbourne, Victoria, Australia.

Smeijsters, H., & van den Hurk, J. (1999). Music therapy helping to work through grief and finding a personal identity. *Journal of Music Therapy, 36*(3), 222–252.

Standley, J. (2000). Music research in medical treatment. In American Music Therapy Association (Ed.), *Effectiveness of music therapy procedures: Documentation of research and clinical practice* (pp. 1– 64). Silver Spring, MD: American Music Therapy Association.

Starr, R. J. (1999). Music therapy in hospice care. *American Journal of Hospice and Palliative Care, 16*(6), 739–742.

Tilden, V. P., Drach, L. L., & Tolle, S. W. (2004). Complementary and alternative therapy use at end-of-life in community settings. *The Journal of Alternative and Complementary Medicine, 10*(5), 811–817.

Trauger-Querry, B., & Haghighi, K. R. (1999). Balancing the focus: Art and music therapy for pain control and symptom management in hospice care. *The Hospice Journal, 14*(1), 25–38.

VanWeelden, K., & Cevasco, A. M. (2007). Repertoire recommendations by music therapists for geriatric clients during singing activities. *Music Therapy Perspectives, 25*, 4–12.

Walker, J., & Adamek, M. (2008). Music therapy in hospice and palliative care. In W. B. Davis, K. E. Gfeller, & M. H. Thaut (Eds.), *An introduction to music therapy theory and practice* (3rd ed., pp. 343–363). Silver Spring, MD: American Music Therapy Association.

Weishaar, K. (1999). The visual life review as a therapeutic art framework with the terminally ill. *The Arts in Psychotherapy, 26*(3), 173–184.

West, T. (1994). Psychological issues in hospice music therapy. *Music Therapy Perspectives, 12*, 117–124.

Whitall, J. (1991). Songs in palliative care: A spouse's last gift. In K. Bruscia (Ed.), *Case studies in music therapy* (pp. 603–610). Phoenixville, PA: Barcelona.

Wlodarczyk, N. (2007). The effect of music therapy on the spirituality of persons in an in-patient hospice unit as measured by self-report. *Journal of Music Therapy, 44*, 113–122.

Wlodarczyk, N. (2008). *The effect of a live music interaction on the stress levels of hospice staff workers during a hospice interdisciplinary team meeting.* Unpublished manuscript.

Wlodarczyk, N. (2009). The use of music and poetry in life review with hospice patients. *Journal of Poetry Therapy, 22*(3), 133–139.

Wlodarczyk, N. (2010). *The effect of a single-session music therapy group intervention for grief resolution on the disenfranchised grief of hospice workers.* Unpublished doctoral dissertation, The Florida State University, Tallahassee, FL.

Worden, J. W. (2009). *Grief counseling and grief therapy: A handbook for the mental health practitioner* (4th ed.). New York: Springer.

Wylie, M., & Blum, R. (1986). Guided imagery and music with hospice patients. *Music Therapy Perspectives, 3*, 25–28.

Wylie, M. E. (1990). A comparison of the effects of old familiar songs, antique objects, historical summaries, and general questions on the reminiscence of nursing home residents. *Journal of Music Therapy, 27*(1), 2–12.

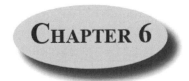

CHAPTER 6

CLINICAL APPLICATIONS FOR PALLIATIVE CARE

FOCUS AREA 1: ADDRESSING PHYSICAL NEEDS WITH MUSIC

Music therapists employ the Iso-Principle—the use of music (1) to carry a person from one emotional state to a more desirable emotional state, (2) to redirect attention from pain or decrease pain perception, and (3) to enhance the pain management regimen by bridging the delivery of medication and the onset of relief. Music therapists can also use the Iso-Principle to contribute to patients' overall comfort by increasing relaxation and decreasing agitation and anxiety.

Music therapists can assist patients in achieving relaxation by using music-assisted progressive muscle relaxation (PMR). Patients can also be taught to use this technique by themselves. Choosing instrumental music can help focus a patient's attention on the task of relaxation by avoiding the distraction of lyrics. Selected music for music-assisted PMR should be steady, soft, and repetitive, and should gradually fade out.

Music can be used as a distraction during the physical discomfort that comes with dressing changes, bathing, turning, blood draws, and other tasks performed by nurses and CNAs. It can also be used to facilitate the timing of breathing exercises. During a patient's final hours, live music can provide comfort to the patient and family. Music can also provide support to other hospice staff members who may be present at the time of death.

Clinical Application 2.1

Target Behavior: Increased relaxation and awareness

Music: Chosen from a variety of genres and time periods; specifically, songs that were popular during the individual's teenage to young adult years. Selected songs should include varying tempos and intensities.

Level 1—General Staff

Directions: Choose several different songs from CDs or MP3 files that have varying tempos and intensities. This activity can be done in a group or individual setting. Start by playing songs that have faster tempos and greater intensity if the individual is agitated or anxious. If the person is already in a relatively calm state, start playing music that is at a moderate tempo. As you progress through playing the songs, choose songs that have less intensity and slower tempos so that you end with a song having a very slow tempo and low intensity. This process should take approximately 30 minutes. Encourage participants to focus on relaxing thoughts paired with deep breathing.

Level 2—Volunteer Musician

Directions: Choose several different songs from your repertoire that have varying tempos and intensities. This activity can be done in a group or individual setting. Start by playing songs that have faster tempos and greater intensity if the individual is agitated or anxious. If the person is already in a relatively calm state, start playing music that is at a moderate tempo. As you progress through playing the songs, choose songs that have less intensity and slower tempos so that you end with a song having a very slow tempo and low intensity. This process should take approximately 30 minutes. Encourage participants to focus on relaxing thoughts paired with deep breathing.

Level 3—Board-Certified Music Therapist

Activity Name: "Iso-Principle Relaxation"

Other Goals Addressed: Increased Quality of Life, Increased Coping, Decreased Perception of Pain

Directions: Choose songs with varying tempos and intensities. This activity can be done in an individual or group setting. Using the Iso-Principle, match the emotional state of the person with the greatest symptoms of need in the group (pain, anxiety, stress, etc.). Using live singing and accompaniment, slowly decrease the intensity and tempo of the music to entrain the participant's emotional or behavioral state. If the individual displays an increase in negative symptoms after showing calmer behavior, match the emotional state again and repeat the process. While the length of this process does vary for each person, typically an individual can experience a lasting, calm emotional state within 30–45 minutes. Assess individual emotional and behavioral states, as well as coping-skill levels for group participants and lead any needed group discussion accordingly.

Clinical Application 2.2

Target Behavior: Increased comfort and relaxation

Music: Instrumental music (without singing/lyrics) that is steady, soft, and repetitive, and gradually fades out.

Progressive Muscle Relaxation Sequence
(Jacobson, 1938; "Progressive Muscle Relaxation," n.d.)

Directions: The purpose of learning the progressive muscle relaxation (PMR) sequence is to develop an awareness of what it physically feels like to be in a calm state, so that same feeling can be elicited by an individual whenever tension, stress, or pain is experienced. However, a history of back problems, serious injury, or muscle spasms could inhibit the success of this exercise. If any group participants have these problems, a physician should be consulted before participation begins.

The PMR sequence is based on two steps: (1) applying tension to muscle groups, and (2) becoming aware of the feeling/sensation present when releasing the tension from the muscles. It is recommended to practice this sequence with participants twice per day for 1 week. Instruct participants to tense the specific muscle for 8 seconds while inhaling their breath. Descriptors of how to tense the muscle may be needed, such as curling the toes of the foot, or pointing the toes while squeezing the thigh for the entire leg sequence. After tensing the muscle for 8 seconds, instruct individuals to release the muscle tension while exhaling their breath and mentally focusing on the feeling of the tension leaving the body. Encourage the group to imagine the pain and tension melting away or floating out of the extremity, such as toes or fingertips. After remaining in a calm state for about 15 seconds, move on to tensing the next muscle group. The order of tensing and releasing muscles is as follows:

Right foot
Right lower leg and foot
Entire right leg
Left foot
Left lower leg and foot
Entire left leg
Right hand
Right forearm and hand
Entire right arm
Left hand
Left forearm and hand
Entire left arm
Abdomen
Chest
Neck and shoulders
Face

After a person feels comfortable with this process, the muscle areas can be grouped together for a shortened version of PMR. There are four muscle groupings: (1) lower limbs; (2) abdomen and chest; (3) arms, shoulders, and neck; and (4) the face. "Cue words" can be spoken by the group leader while exhaling and releasing tension such as "relax," "stay calm," "everything is okay," etc. Eventually, hearing the cue word will automatically elicit a calm behavioral state and, therefore, a calm mental state.

Level 1—General Staff

Directions: Follow the PMR sequence and play recorded music from CDs or MP3 files to assist with the process.

Level 2—Volunteer Musician

Directions: Follow the PMR sequence and play live instrumental music, if appropriate, or recorded music from CDs or MP3 files to assist with the process.

Level 3—Board-Certified Music Therapist

Activity Name: "Progressive Muscle Relaxation"

Other Goals Addressed: Increased Quality of Life, Increased Coping

Directions: Follow the PMR sequence and play live instrumental music, if appropriate, or recorded music from CDs or MP3 files to assist with the process. Assess behavioral responses during the PMR sequence to identify individuals who are struggling with the process or getting stuck during a specific part of the PMR exercise. After finishing the sequence, address any emotional or physical issues that could be preventing the individual from fully completing the PMR sequence through music therapy counseling.

Clinical Application 2.3

Target Behavior: Decreased perception of pain

Music: Music most preferred by each individual. Consult with family members if needed to determine the individual's preferred music.

Level 1—General Staff

Directions: Choose several different songs from CDs or MP3 files from each person's most preferred and known music. Create a compilation of songs that will be very engaging for individuals when they are experiencing pain. Pain can be experienced during procedures such as bath time, dressing changes, or needle insertions. Consult with the nursing staff to determine when procedures are scheduled for the individual. Approximately 10 minutes before the procedure is to begin, start playing the compilation of songs. Continue playing the music throughout the procedure and for 10–15 minutes after the procedure ends. The goal is to distract the patient from the painful procedure by engaging him/her with the music.

Level 2—Volunteer Musician

Directions: Choose several different songs from your repertoire that are favored by participants. Create a compilation of songs that will be engaging for individuals when they are experiencing pain. Pain can be experienced during procedures such as bath time, dressing changes, or needle insertions. Consult with the nursing staff to determine when procedures are scheduled for each individual. Start playing the compilation of songs approximately 10 minutes before the procedure is scheduled to begin. Continue playing the music throughout the procedure and for 10–15 minutes after the procedure ends. The goal is to distract the patient from the painful procedure by engaging him/her with the music.

Level 3—Board-Certified Music Therapist

Activity Name: "Music for Procedural Support"

Other Goals Addressed: Increased Coping with Procedures, Increased Relaxation, Increased Quality of Life

Directions: Consult with nursing staff to find out when painful procedures are scheduled for the individual, such as dressing changes, baths, or needle insertions. If you have not previously seen the individual and need to assess his/her preferred music, set up a time to establish rapport and identify his/her music preference before engaging in this intervention. On the day of the procedure, arrive 10 minutes before the procedure is scheduled to begin. Using the Iso-Principle, sing live music with accompaniment to assist the patient/client in achieving the most relaxed state possible. Once the painful procedure begins, continue using the Iso-Principle to match the emotional and behavioral state of the individual throughout the procedure. Use the most familiar and engaging music for the patient during the procedure to allow him/her to participate/engage with the music. When the procedure is complete, continue using the Iso-Principle to return the individual to a calm resting state. For patients with extreme anxiety about the procedure, you may also use techniques described in Clinical Application 2.4 for several sessions leading up to the day of the scheduled procedure.

Clinical Application 2.4

Target Behavior: Increased relaxation during anxiety-producing or painful procedures

Music: Music most preferred by each individual. Consult with family members if needed to determine the patient/client preferred music.

Self-Guided Visualization for Relaxation

Directions: Allow the individual to choose a relaxing place to imagine in their minds.

Level 1—General Staff

Directions: Choose several different songs from CDs or MP3 files from each person's most preferred and known music. Create a compilation of songs that will be very engaging for individuals when they are experiencing pain. Pain can be experienced during procedures such as bath time, dressing changes, or needle insertions. Consult with the nursing staff to determine when procedures are scheduled for the individual. Meet with the individual for several days leading up to the procedure to practice relaxation exercises paired with music. Lead the patient/client in a self-guided visualization to promote relaxation. The same music should be played in the same order throughout each visualization exercise. On the day of the procedure, start playing the compilation of songs approximately 10 minutes before the scheduled procedure is to begin. Continue playing the music throughout the procedure and for 10–15 minutes after the procedure ends. The goal of this intervention is to assist patients in achieving a relaxed state as soon as they hear the music and to distract them from painful procedures by engaging them with the music.

Level 2—Volunteer Musician

Directions: Choose several different songs from your repertoire that are each person's most preferred and known music. Create a compilation of songs that will be engaging for individuals when they are experiencing pain. Pain can be experienced during procedures such as bath time, dressing changes, or needle insertions. Consult with the nursing staff to determine when procedures are scheduled for each individual. Meet with the individual for several days leading up to the procedure to practice relaxation exercises paired with music. Lead the patient/client in a self-guided visualization to promote relaxation. The same music should be played in the same order throughout each visualization exercise. On the day of the procedure, start playing the compilation of songs approximately 10 minutes before the procedure is to begin. Continue playing the music throughout the procedure and for 10–15 minutes after the procedure ends. The goal of this intervention is to assist patients in achieving a relaxed state as soon as they hear the music and to distract them from painful procedures by engaging them with the music.

Level 3—Board-Certified Music Therapist

Activity Name: "Music and Imagery-Elicited Relaxation"

Other Goals Addressed: Quality of Life

Directions: Schedule at least three music therapy sessions before the anxiety-producing or painful procedure is scheduled to occur. During these preliminary music therapy sessions, identify the most preferred music for relaxation for the individual. Lead the patient/client through a music imagery session using the individual's preferred imagery. Play the songs in the same order for every preliminary session while the individual is describing his/her relaxing imagery. Focus on deep breathing and awareness of how relaxation feels throughout the body. If the patient becomes agitated or "blocked" during the imagery time, use verbal counseling techniques paired with the Iso-Principle to return the individual to a relaxed and calm behavioral state. On the day of the procedure, approximately 10 minutes before the procedure is to begin, start playing the individual's preferred relaxation songs in the same order played during the preliminary sessions. Continue playing the music throughout the procedure. When the procedure is complete, continue using the Iso-Principle to return the individual to a calm resting state.

FOCUS AREA 2: ADDRESSING PSYCHOSOCIAL NEEDS WITH MUSIC

Music can decrease confusion by bringing familiarity into the environment with patient-preferred music. Communication aids, such as laminated visuals, choice wheels, or dice, can increase communication opportunities and allow patients to make song choices. Music, such as bedside singing, can be used as a structural support to promote positive interactions between family members. Songwriting, lyric analysis, and life review projects can be used to communicate with loved ones, leave a tangible product for living family members, decrease feelings of isolation, and address anticipatory grief (feelings of grief leading up to the death).

Clinical Application 2.5

Target Behavior: Increased emotional awareness

Music: Music most preferred by the individual. Consult with family members if needed to determine the individual's preferred music.

Level 1—General Staff

Directions: Ask individuals to write their life story in only five sentences on a piece of paper or white board. When given only five possible sentences, participants must think about the most valuable aspects of their lives. Provide individuals with some options of recorded music and have them choose a song that best represents the intended emotional content of their life story. Play the recording of the song while reading the life story to enhance the emotional content of the story. Let the song play through to the end and invite reactions, if desired.

Level 2—Volunteer Musician

Directions: Ask individuals to write their life story in only five sentences on a piece of paper or white board. When given only five possible sentences, participants must think about the most valuable aspects of their own life. Provide individuals with some song options from your repertoire and have them choose a song that best represents the intended emotional content of their life story. Play the song while reading the life story to enhance the emotional content of the story. Let the song play through to the end and invite reactions, if desired.

Level 3—Board-Certified Music Therapist

Activity Name: "Life Story to Music"

Other Goals Addressed: Increased Sense of Self, Increased Coping, Increased Quality of Life

Directions: Ask individuals to write their life story in only five sentences on a piece of paper or white board. When given only five possible sentences, participants must think about the most valuable aspects of their own life. During this activity, life events may be recalled that require emotional and cognitive processing by the individual. If this occurs, use counseling techniques to help the patient process the life events in a healthy way. Provide individuals with some song options from your repertoire and have them choose a song that best represents the intended emotional content of their life story. Play the song while reading the life story to enhance the emotional content of their story. Let the song play through to the end and invite reactions and discussion. This activity can also be done with improvised music.

Clinical Application 2.6

Target Behavior: Increased emotional awareness

Music: Music most preferred by each individual. Consult with family members if needed to determine the individual's preferred music.

Level 1—General Staff

Directions: Choose several different songs from CDs or MP3 files that have themes relating to life review, such as "My Way," "I Still Haven't Found What I'm Looking For," or "I'll Fly Away." Play the songs that seem appropriate for the individual's current mood state. Encourage the patient/client to talk about how he/she feels when hearing the words to the songs.

Level 2—Volunteer Musician

Directions: Make a performance list from your repertoire of songs that have lyrics relating to life review, such as "My Way," "I Still Haven't Found What I'm Looking For," or "I'll Fly Away." Play the songs that seem appropriate for the individual's current mood state. Encourage the patient/client to talk about how he/she feels when hearing the words to the songs.

Level 3—Board-Certified Music Therapist

Activity Name: "Songwriting for Healing"

Other Goals Addressed: Decreased Anxiety, Increased Coping, Reminiscence, Increased Quality of Life

Directions: Choose songs with thematic content about life review, such as "My Way," "I Still Haven't Found What I'm Looking For," or "I'll Fly Away." After playing the songs, encourage discussion regarding the emotions that are evoked when the individual reflects on his/her life. During this conversation, life events may be elicited that require emotional and cognitive processing by the individual. If this occurs, use counseling techniques to help the patient process the life events. Assess the individual's emotional state and coping-skill abilities while involved in the discussion with the patient/client. After establishing the emotional needs of the patient, ask the individual if he/she would like to write a song summarizing the thoughts brought up in the discussion. Choose a style of music preferred by the patient. The song may be an original composition or a parody of an existing melody. After writing the song to reflect the current emotional state of the patient/client, play the song for the individual as an affirmation of his/her strengths and accomplishments. The song may be used in subsequent sessions as a starting point for further counseling of grief processing, if needed.

Clinical Application 2.7

Target Behavior: Increased coping

Music: Music most preferred by each individual. Consult with family members if needed to determine the individual's preferred music.

Level 1—General Staff

Directions: Have several different songs from CDs or MP3 files that individuals can listen to. Invite the patients/clients to identify a song that they feel represents them well. If an individual cannot identify a song, suggest several songs that could reflect the personality and character of the individual. After listening to each song, discuss whether or not that song would be a good choice for the patient/client as his/her "life song." Once the song is chosen, write a letter to family members from the individual, sharing the song choice and the reason why that song was chosen to represent their loved one. The letter may also share a story or memory that the patient associates with the chosen song. Another option is to create a scrapbook combining pictures, stories, and meaningful song lyrics that can be given as a gift to family members/loved ones.

Level 2—Volunteer Musician

Directions: Make a performance list from your repertoire of songs of several different types of genres and songs. Invite the patients/clients to identify a life song that they feel represents them well. If an individual cannot identify a song, suggest several songs that could reflect the personality and character of the individual. After listening to each song, discuss whether or not that song would be a good choice for the patient/client as his/her "life song." Once the song is chosen, write a letter to family members from the individual sharing the song choice and the reason why that song was chosen to represent their loved one. The letter may also share a story or memory that the patient associates with the chosen song. Another option is to create a scrapbook combining pictures, stories, and meaningful song lyrics that can be given as a gift to family members/loved ones.

Level 3—Board-Certified Music Therapist

Activity Name: "Living Legacy"

Other Goals Addressed: Increased Quality of Life, Caregiver Bonding, Increased Awareness of Emotion

Directions: A "Living Legacy" project is a multimedia representation of the patient's life, usually created over the course of several focused sessions. If the patient/client desires family involvement, invite family members/loved ones to attend music therapy sessions with the individual. During these sessions, identify important events and characteristics of the patient and his/her life. Write down stories and memories that are discussed during the sessions. Encourage the patient and family to bring pictures of the patient's life to include in the Living Legacy project. Discuss what the patient feels is his/her legacy to leave to future generations and write a song that accurately reflects the patient's wishes. Use the stylistic preference of the patient when composing the song. The song can be an original composition or a parody of an existing favorite melody of the patient. After the patient hears and approves this Living Legacy song, record the song as a gift to the family. The patient can sing the song to the family, or you can sing for the recording. Have the patient present the song as a gift to the family, along with any accompanying scrapbooks with pictures, stories, and songs written for family members. Another possibility is a video project incorporating old home movies and new videos of the patient and family in music therapy sessions.

Clinical Application 2.8

Target Behavior: Increased life satisfaction and rejuvenation

Music: Chosen from a variety of genres and from different time periods as preferred by the individual.

Level 1—General Staff

Directions: Choose several different songs from CDs or MP3 files that have themes relating to feeling down, such as "I'm So Lonesome I Could Cry," "One for My Baby," or "Pass Me Not." Play the songs for the individual and then encourage him/her to discuss how he/she relates to the feelings expressed in the songs. The goal is for the songs to provide a starting point for discussion.

Level 2—Volunteer Musician

Directions: Make a performance list from your repertoire of songs that have lyrics relating to feeling down, such as "I'm So Lonesome I Could Cry," "One for My Baby," or "Pass Me Not." Play the songs for the individual and then encourage him/her to discuss how he/she relates to the feelings expressed in the songs. The goal is for the songs to provide a starting point for discussion.

Level 3—Board-Certified Music Therapist

Activity Name: "Lyric Analysis for Depression"

Other Goals Addressed: Decreased Anxiety, Increased Coping

Directions: Choose a song with content about feeling depressed or lonely, such as "I'm So Lonesome I Could Cry," "One for My Baby," or "Pass Me Not." Lead a lyric analysis of the selected songs, focusing on validation and coping strategies. Assess individual emotional states and coping-skill levels for the individual and lead the discussion accordingly. Choose a song with positive coping skills reflected in the lyrics, such as "Steal Away" or "It Is Well with My Soul" and lead a lyric analysis discussing positive coping strategies. Assist the patient in identifying coping skills that can be implemented in his/her daily life.

FOCUS AREA 3: ADDRESSING SPIRITUAL NEEDS WITH MUSIC

For many individuals, there is an obvious connection between the dying process, spirituality, and music. Music therapy can "bring church to the patient" when the patient is no longer able to leave home and thus provide an opportunity for worship, prayer, or meditation. Songwriting and lyric analysis can be paired with a favorite scripture. Lyric analysis and reflection can be used to promote feelings of acceptance and reconciliation. The music therapist can also assist patients in planning the music for their memorial services, thus allowing them a sense of control over how they will be remembered.

Clinical Application 2.9

Target Behavior: Increased relaxation

Music: Instrumental music that promotes the creation of a relaxing and comforting environment, incorporating environmental sounds such as rain, ocean waves, etc. The environmental sounds must be considered relaxing and comforting by the patient.

Level 1—General Staff

Directions: Create a "sacred space" for meditation using instruments, voices, props, and environmental sounds such as rain, ocean waves, etc. *Sacred space* is a term used by hospice chaplains to describe an environment structured to facilitate meditation, relaxation, or prayer. To create this environment, close off the room to external noise and distractions, and instruct the patient to close his/her eyes if comfortable or to focus on deep breathing. Play recorded background music that the patient/client prefers to facilitate a relaxing environment. Encourage the individual to meditate, relax, or pray.

Level 2—Volunteer Musician

Directions: Create a "sacred space" for meditation using instruments, voices, props, and environmental sounds such as rain, ocean waves, etc. *Sacred space* is a term used by hospice chaplains to describe an environment structured to facilitate meditation, relaxation, or prayer. To create this environment, close off the room to external noise and distractions, and instruct the patient to close his/her eyes if comfortable or to focus on deep breathing. Play instruments you have available that will facilitate a relaxing environment. Encourage the individual to meditate, relax, or pray.

Level 3—Board-Certified Music Therapist

Activity Name: "My Sacred Space"
This activity can lead to patients' increased relaxation as well as facilitate their meditative thoughts (Foxglove & Tyas, 2000).

Other Goals Addressed: Spiritual Support, Increased Quality of Life, Increased Coping

Directions: Create a "sacred space" for meditation using instruments, voices, props, and the environmental sounds such as rain, ocean waves, etc. *Sacred space* is a term used by hospice chaplains to describe an environment structured to facilitate meditation, relaxation, or prayer. This environment is created by closing off the room to external noise and distractions and having the patient close his/her eyes if comfortable or to focus on deep breathing. Assist in creating a meditative environment by using instruments that mimic sounds such as light rain or ocean waves. Use instruments such as rain sticks, thunder tubes, and ocean drums to mimic the sound of rain, thunder, and the ocean. You may also use improvisational guitar or keyboard sounds. Help the individual achieve maximum relaxation, meditation, or prayer by identifying and processing any issues that could be getting in the way of this experience. Once those issues have been addressed, offer to lead the patient/client through his/her preferred relaxation, meditation, or prayer time and provide support as needed.

Clinical Application 2.10

Target Behavior: Increased coping and acceptance

Music: Chosen from a variety of genres and from different time periods as preferred by the individual.

Level 1—General Staff

Directions: Ask patients/clients if they have thought about music they want played at their funeral, if they are planning to have a funeral. If the individual has some favorite songs, specific arrangements/recordings can be chosen after listening to several different options. If the individual has not thought about music for his/her funeral, play several different selections of songs that seem appropriate based on the patient/client's value system, life story, and personality. The purpose of this conversation is to open the door to the topic and allow the patient to begin thinking about the music that he/she would want played at the funeral. If an emotional response results from this conversation, refer the patient/client to the appropriate trained staff member to process the issues appropriately.

Level 2—Volunteer Musician

Directions: Ask patients/clients if they have thought about music they want played at their funeral, if they are planning to have a funeral. If you are willing to play live music at the funeral, you can play arrangements from your repertoire for possible funeral song options. Otherwise, if the individual has some favorite songs, specific arrangements/recordings can be chosen after listening to several different options. If the individual has not thought about music for his/her funeral, play several different selections of songs that seem appropriate based on the patient/client's value system, life story, and personality. As you progress through the song choices, note which features the individual likes/dislikes to help you make further choices. After the individual has chosen the songs he/she would like to have played at the funeral, encourage him/her to share the selections with family members or loved ones who will be responsible for funeral arrangements. If an emotional response results from this conversation, refer the patient/client to the appropriate trained staff member to process the issues appropriately.

Level 3—Board-Certified Music Therapist

Activity Name: "Funeral Preparation"

Other Goals Addressed: Quality of Life, Autonomy/Choice-Making

Directions: The process of funeral planning may take several sessions, depending on the acceptance level and needs of the patient. Ask patients/clients if they have thought about music they want played at their funeral, if they are planning to have a funeral. If you are willing to play live music at the funeral, you can play arrangements from your repertoire for possible funeral song options. Otherwise, if the individual has some favorite songs, specific arrangements/recordings can be chosen after listening to several different options. If the individual has not thought about music for his/her funeral, play several different selections of songs that seem appropriate based on the patient/client's spiritual background, value system, life story, and personality. As you progress through the song choices, note which features the individual likes/dislikes to help you make further choices. After the individual has chosen the songs he/she would like to have played at the funeral, encourage him/her to share the selections with family members or loved ones who will be responsible for funeral arrangements. If an emotional response results from this conversation, address the patient's feelings and concerns through music therapy counseling techniques.

Clinical Application 2.11

Target Behavior: Increased spiritual support

Music: Spiritual music that is preferred by the individual.

Level 1—General Staff

Directions: After identifying the type of spiritual music preferred by the individual, choose several songs that have supportive themes in the lyrics. Play the recordings (MP3 or CDs) of the songs and provide a copy of the lyrics for the individual to follow along with while listening to the song. After each song, invite discussion of the lyrics and themes conveyed in the song. If an emotional response results from this conversation, refer the patient/client to the appropriate trained staff member to process the issues appropriately.

Level 2—Volunteer Musician

Directions: After identifying the type of spiritual music preferred by the individual, choose several songs from your repertoire that have supportive themes in the lyrics. Play the songs and provide a copy of the lyrics for the individual to follow along with while listening to the song. After each song, invite discussion of the lyrics and themes conveyed in the song. If an emotional response results from this conversation, refer the patient/client to the appropriate trained staff member to process the issues appropriately.

Level 3—Board-Certified Music Therapist

Activity Name: "Spiritual Support Analysis"

Other Goals Addressed: Increased Coping, Increased Quality of Life

Directions: After identifying the type of spiritual music preferred by the individual, play the songs and lead a lyric analysis, focusing on those songs that have supportive or uplifting themes. Encourage the patient/client to identify sources of spiritual strength and target any areas of spiritual distress. If an emotional response results from this conversation, address the patient's feelings and concerns through music therapy counseling techniques. If the patient's spiritual distress is significant, refer a chaplain for an assessment or co-visit.

Clinical Application 2.12

Target Behavior: Increased spiritual awareness

Music: Spiritual music that is preferred by the individual.

Level 1—General Staff

Directions: A *spiritual footprint* is a patient's unique and individual story of his/her spiritual journey throughout his/her lifetime. Encourage individuals to share their spiritual journey, writing down all salient events from their past to form their own unique "spiritual footprint." After identifying the type of spiritual music preferred by the individual, choose several songs from CDs or MP3s that the patient feels relate to his/her spiritual footprint and listen to them together. Engage the patient in conversation as appropriate. If an emotional response results from this activity, refer a chaplain or appropriate staff member.

Level 2—Volunteer Musician

Directions: A *spiritual footprint* is a patient's unique and individual story of his/her spiritual journey throughout his/her lifetime. Encourage individuals to share their spiritual journey, writing down all salient events from their past to form their own unique "spiritual footprint." After identifying the type of spiritual music preferred by the individual, choose several songs from your repertoire that the patient feels relate to his/her spiritual footprint and play them for the patient. Engage the patient in conversation as appropriate. If an emotional response results from this activity, refer a chaplain or appropriate staff member.

Level 3—Board-Certified Music Therapist

Activity Name: "Spiritual Footprint"

Other Goals Addressed: Increased Coping, Increased Quality of Life

Directions: A *spiritual footprint* is a patient's unique and individual story of his/her spiritual journey throughout his/her lifetime. Encourage individuals to share their spiritual journey, writing down all salient events from their past to form their own unique "spiritual footprint." After identifying the type of spiritual music preferred by the individual, choose several songs from your repertoire that have themes in the lyrics that relate well to the individual's spiritual footprint. Insert the songs into the spiritual footprint at the appropriate places. The spiritual footprint may be recorded in audio or visual format to be shared with the family, if the patient desires. If an emotional response results from this activity, address the patient's feelings and concerns through music therapy counseling techniques. If the patient's spiritual distress is significant, refer a chaplain for an assessment or co-visit.

FOCUS AREA 4: ADDRESSING BEREAVEMENT NEEDS WITH MUSIC

Through one-to-one sessions or groups, music therapists can address issues of grief through many of the music therapy techniques that have already been discussed in this unit. Possible bereavement topics include coping skills, planning for the future, and teaching family members to use music at home for grief support. Reminiscence activities using the patient's favorite music can also help to say goodbye and promote feelings of closure. Living legacy projects are also a positive and pleasurable way to remember loved ones.

Clinical Application 2.13

Target Behavior: Increased grief support

Music: Music most preferred by the individual.

Level 1—General Staff

Directions: The following worksheet titled "My Mood Music" is used with bereaved persons to teach them to use their own music at home for grief support. The worksheet lists various mood states that a grieving person may feel. To introduce the worksheet, have many different songs from CDs available that convey different emotional states for patients to listen to during this exercise. Keep in mind that because music preference is very individualized, a song that might encourage one person could make another person feel frustrated. Help the individual identify music that has a positive impact on him/her when feeling each of the different mood states listed on the My Mood Music worksheet. If emotional needs arise during this process, refer the individual to the appropriate trained staff member to process the issues.

Level 2—Volunteer Musician

Directions: The following worksheet titled "My Mood Music" is used with bereaved persons to teach them to use their own music at home for grief support. The worksheet lists various mood states that a grieving person may feel. To introduce the worksheet, have many different songs available from your repertoire that convey different emotional states for patients to listen to during this exercise. Keep in mind that because music preference is very individualized, a song that might encourage one person could make another person feel frustrated. Help the individual identify music that has a positive impact on him/her when feeling each of the different mood states listed on the My Mood Music worksheet. If emotional needs arise during this process, refer the individual to the appropriate trained staff member to process the issues.

Level 3—Board-Certified Music Therapist

Activity Name: "My Mood Music"

Other Goals Addressed: Increased Coping, Increased Quality of Life

Directions: The following worksheet titled "My Mood Music" is used with bereaved persons to teach them to use their own music at home for grief support. The worksheet lists various mood states that a grieving person may feel. Lead a discussion that describes the way music can affect mood and how choosing music for different mood states can give grieving persons some control over their emotional state. Assist the individual in filling out the worksheet to identify music that has a positive impact on him/her when feeling each of the different mood states listed. During this process, emotional needs may arise that should be addressed through music therapy counseling techniques. Process the issues that surface with the individual as they arise.

My Mood Music	
When I am…	**I'll listen to…**
Sad	
Mellow	
Excited	
Restless	
Alone with thoughts	
Content	
Needing to relax	
Feeling hopeful	
Lonely	
Exercising	
With friends	
On a road trip	
Thinking about him/her	
Dancing shamelessly	
Trying to fall asleep	
Avoiding	
Cleaning	
Meditating/praying	
Trying to wake up	
Thankful	

Clinical Application 2.14

Target Behavior: Increased grief support

Music: Music most preferred by the individual.

Level 1—General Staff

Directions: Ask the individual to select a song that sends a message to a loved one, or a song that illustrates the way he/she would like to be remembered. Some song examples are "I Will Remember You" by Sarah McLachlan, "My Heart Will Go On" by Celine Dion, or "Unforgettable" by Nat King Cole. Play through as many recordings of songs as necessary for the individual to find the most meaningful song for him/her. Once the "right" song has been selected, offer to invite the person to whom the song is being "sent" to hear you play the song. If this song is a gift in memory of a deceased loved one, create a special moment to play the song as a gift, with any accompanying messages the individual wants to convey. If emotional needs arise during this process, refer the individual to the appropriate trained staff member to process the issues appropriately.

Level 2—Volunteer Musician

Directions: Create a song list from your repertoire of songs that are appropriate "Message Songs." Ask the individual to select a song from the list that sends a message to a loved one, or a song that illustrates the way he/she would like to be remembered. Play through as many songs as necessary for the individual to find the most meaningful song for him/her. Once the "right" song has been selected, offer to invite the person to whom the song is being "sent" to hear you play the song. If this song is a gift in memory of a deceased loved one, create a special moment to play the song as a gift, with any accompanying messages the individual wants to convey. If emotional needs arise during this process, refer the individual to the appropriate trained staff member to process the issues appropriately.

Level 3—Board-Certified Music Therapist

Activity Name: "Song Message"

Other Goals Addressed: Increased Quality of Life, Increased Bonding

Directions: Ask the individual to select a song that sends a message to a loved one, or a song that illustrates the way he/she would like to be remembered. Some song examples are "I Will Remember You" by Sarah McLachlan, "My Heart Will Go On" by Celine Dion, or "Unforgettable" by Nat King Cole. Play through as many songs as necessary for the individual to find the most meaningful song for him/her. Once the "right" song has been selected, offer to invite the person to whom the song is being "sent" to hear you play the song. If this song is a gift in memory of a deceased loved one, create a special moment to play the song as a gift, with any accompanying messages the individual wants to convey. During this process, emotional needs may arise that will need to be addressed through music therapy counseling techniques. Process the issues that surface with the individual as they arise.

Clinical Application 2.15

Target Behavior: Increased grief support

Music: Drums of various types and sizes.

Level 1—General Staff &
Level 2—Volunteer Musician

Directions: This activity can be done in a group setting or with individuals of any age. Gather as many drums as needed so that all participants have their own drum. If using very large gathering drums, multiple people can share the same drum. Invite whoever is most comfortable to start playing a rhythm on a drum. Explain to participants that when they are ready, they can join in with their own rhythm on top of the existing rhythm being played. Encourage individuals to listen carefully to the sounds in the room. This drumming time can allow individuals to express their feelings in a constructive way to release any negative feelings, such as frustration and anger, that they might be experiencing during the grief process. If emotional needs arise during this process, refer the patient/client to the appropriate trained staff member to process the issues appropriately.

Level 3—Board-Certified Music Therapist

Activity Name: "Drum It Out"

Other Goals Addressed: Increased Coping, Decreased Negative Behaviors, Increased Quality of Life

Directions: This activity can be done in a group setting or with individuals of any age. Gather as many drums as needed so that all participants have their own drum. If using very large gathering drums, multiple people can share the same drum. Invite whoever is most comfortable to start playing a rhythm on a drum. Explain to participants that when they are ready, they can join in with their own rhythm on top of the existing rhythm being played. Encourage individuals to listen carefully to the sounds in the room. Assist the group in making transfers to the grief process (i.e., nobody was playing quite the same rhythm; no two individuals' grief is the same, everyone grieves differently, etc.). This drumming time can allow individuals to express their feelings in a constructive way to release any negative feelings, such as frustration and anger, that they might be experiencing during the grief process. Another variation is to divide the group in half and teach a simple rhythm to each smaller group to play together. Participants who are able can take turns standing in front of the group and "directing," using simple hand motions such as raising/lowering hands to indicate the group should get louder/softer. Engage in a discussion about how it feels to lead the group, for example, experiencing feelings of control, etc. During this process, emotional needs may arise that will need to be addressed through music therapy counseling techniques. Process the issues that surface with the individuals as they arise.

REFERENCES

Foxglove, T., & Tyas, B. (2000). Using music as a spiritual tool in palliative care. *European Journal of Palliative Care, 7*(2), 63–65.

Jacobson, E. (1938). *Progressive relaxation.* Chicago: University of Chicago Press.

Progressive mental relaxation. (n.d.) *A guide to psychology and its practice.* Retrieved from http://www.guidetopsychology.com/pmr.htm

Unit III
Music Therapy
for
Health and Wellness

CHAPTER 7

INTRODUCTION TO HEALTH AND WELLNESS AND MUSIC THERAPY

You know, I used to dread my morning walks, but now I just put on my headset and go. I think nothing of it listening to my favorite music, and you know, it seems I am finished with my three miles in a fraction of the time. —Mr. K.

I'm going to take up the guitar 'cause I've always wanted to play one and now there's time to practice. —Mrs. A.

HEALTH AND WELLNESS

Wellness, which is often paired with health—as in "health and wellness," is considered to be the balance of mind, body, and spirit that results in one's general sense of well-being. The American Music Therapy Association (2005) has set forth standards of clinical practice in the area of wellness and defines this area of music therapy practice as "the specialized use of music to enhance quality of life, to maximize well-being and potential, and to increase self-awareness in individuals seeking music therapy services." Wellness programs include proactive interventions designed to maintain participants' present physical, cognitive, and emotional health and to prevent future illnesses. Such programs are frequently offered by hospitals, community organizations such as YMCAs or senior centers, and private or public health clubs.

Wellness programs are most often a combination of educational and organizational activities designed to support behaviors that are conducive to good health. Common wellness activities are related to nutritional awareness, physical fitness, stress management, cognitive fitness, as well as emotional and social support. Wellness programs cover the lifespan; however, wellness activities are especially important to older adults, who upon retirement often become less active.

Functional disabilities and physical impairments increase with age; therefore, vigorous efforts toward disease prevention and health promotion for seniors are warranted. Chronic diseases and disabling conditions exert personal and economic burdens on older adults. Age-related diseases and conditions result in diminished quality of life and the associated costs of long-term illnesses. Approximately 80% of older Americans are living with at least one chronic condition, and 50% have at least two (Administration on Aging, 2008). Wellness activities can do much to counteract the natural effects of the aging process. Such activities empower older persons to adopt healthy behaviors and thus better enable them to properly manage chronic conditions. Many of the illnesses, disabilities, and deaths that accompany chronic diseases are avoidable through preventative measures associated with wellness programs. In addition, wellness programs are cost effective because they are less expensive than the healthcare required for individuals who are ill.

HISTORY OF WELLNESS PROGRAMS FOR OLDER ADULTS

Until the 1980s, older adults were not considered age-appropriate for wellness programs (Walker, 1991). They were generally viewed as past the age at which preventative measures would be effective. It became increasingly clear, however, that illness-based care alone was not sufficient in maintaining the health of older adults. In 1988, the United States Surgeon General convened the Workshop of Health Promotion and Aging to assess current knowledge on health promotion among older adults and to make recommendations for policy, service, education, and research in wellness programs for senior citizens (Walker, 1991). Governmental initiatives played an important role in the development of community-based wellness programs for seniors. Such programs have become popular among seniors, as well as proven cost effective in preventing age-related illnesses (Benson & McDevitt, 1989).

As medical technology has advanced, so have the costs of healthcare. The promotion of wellness programs for older adults has been prompted, in part, by the rising costs of long-term care, particularly those associated with residential care in assisted living and nursing facilities. Research has also played a role in the promotion of wellness programs for older adults. Researchers have found a relationship between physical, nutritional, and emotional health and the age-related illnesses that often result in seniors being admitted to long-term care facilities (Gutt, 1996). The longer older adults remain healthy, the fewer years they spend in expensive nursing homes, which ultimately puts less stress on healthcare systems.

Other factors that have played a role in the promotion of wellness programs for older adults have been the popularization of fitness programs in general, and an increasing acceptance of holistic medicine. Health was once viewed as simply the absence of physical illness. Over the years, the concept of health has become increasingly multidimensional and now includes mental, social, and spiritual aspects as well as physical. Older adults have become more tuned to the importance of emotional and spiritual health and have embraced components of wellness programs that address those personal needs (Ghetti, Hama, & Woolrich, 2008). Music therapy is one wellness activity that includes goals directed toward all aspects of health.

MUSIC AND WELLNESS

Music has the potential to enhance all areas of wellness programs. Music can serve as a motivator and reward for engaging in many activities that promote general wellness. These activities are generally directed toward physical or cognitive functioning, socialization, and lifelong learning. Music, because of its pervasiveness, universal appeal, and flexibility in terms of tempo, complexity, and genres, is particularly suited to accompany numerous physical, cognitive, and social activities. Music can be used to provide structure for physical and social activities, to provide emotional support, and to promote lifelong learning. Music therapy interventions have been employed to decrease arousal due to stress (Bittman et al., 2005; Pelletier, 2004), to facilitate adherence to physical rehabilitation exercises (Johnson, Otto, & Clair,

2001), to improve balance and gait of older persons (Hamburg & Clair, 2003), to reduce sleep disturbances in the elderly (Johnson, 2003; Lai & Good, 2005; Mornhinweg & Voignier, 1995), and to reduce symptoms of depression in the elderly (Hanser, 1990; Hanser & Thompson, 1994). Strategies for lifelong learning, such as instrumental playing, have been used to facilitate physical rehabilitation (Zelazny, 2001) and to improve working memory in older adults (Bugos, 2007).

Most individuals of any age enjoy some style of music, whether just listening to the music or actively engaging in music making. In addition to its general appeal, music is also highly flexible in regard to style, age-appropriateness, or type (instrumental vs. vocal). Because of its versatility and pervasiveness in our social environments (stores, restaurants, sports events, etc.), music is a useful medium for promoting and maintaining engagement in health-related activities. Music serves easily as a facilitator of socialization and physical activity—both important components of general wellness. Few individuals exercise or dance without music. Attending musical events is a realistic and opportune way to encourage older adults to engage in community activities.

Active engagement (music making) and receptive participation (music listening) in music both have the potential to impact one's health. Instrument playing has been shown to increase manual dexterity and range of motion, while music listening has been shown to improve mood states and increase physical endurance (Clair & Memmott, 2008). Participating in music lessons has even been shown to reduce stress and improve mood (Grape, Sandgren, Hansson, Ericson, & Theorell, 2003). Such data provide the rationale for lifelong learning in music.

LIFELONG LEARNING AND MUSIC

Lifelong learning is the pursuit of knowledge at any age and in any context. The term implies that learning is not confined to childhood or to schools, nor to the pursuit of a degree. Instead, learning occurs throughout life and in a wide range of places and situations. Learning is open to all citizens for either personal or professional reasons, or for personal development, social inclusion, and personal fulfillment or enjoyment. Because of changes in contemporary society, particularly advances in technology that impact the daily lives of all citizens, education need not be confined to the early years of life. Opportunities for learning offered to individuals can sustain them throughout their lives.

Lifelong learning tends to be learner-centered in that learning is generally initiated and structured by the learner. Lifelong learners are generally self-directed and engage in learning tasks based on their needs, interests, or desires. Contemporary technology has contributed much to lifelong learning. Computers have broken the restraints of time and place for learning and have made learning convenient and flexible for older learners. Older adults who are homebound or who require instructional adaptations such as large print, amplification, or additional time to master new skills can easily be accommodated through e-learning. Computers, electronic music games, and other e-learning tools have made music education flexible, fun, and accessible for independent study.

Music can play an important role in lifelong learning programs for older adults. Learning a new instrument, taking singing lessons, or making music with others are opportunities that can be easily instituted in assisted living and nursing facilities to engage the mind, promote socialization, and provide adults with a sense of accomplishment. Technological advances in music now allow individuals an opportunity to perform music regardless of their physical or cognitive abilities. A plethora of adaptive devices for persons with physical disabilities are now available for acoustic or electronic instruments, as well as equipment for recording and listening to music. Music can also be adapted for either passive or active involvement.

Many older adults were involved with music in their younger years and wish to maintain their musical interests and skills, while other adults never had the opportunity to study music but wish to in retirement. With the right teacher, music lessons can provide older learners with an enjoyable and relaxing leisure skill. Most teachers of older adults do not put the same demands to practice on their older learners as they do on their young students. These teachers understand that music is not going to become a career for their older learners; consequently, many music teachers enjoy working with older adults because they can adopt a "music for fun" approach to their teaching. Many older adults, however, are quite serious about their music lessons. The ability to develop musical skills remains throughout the lifespan. Gibbons (1983) found that the older adults' abilities to acquire musical skills remain strong into their 90s.

Music ensembles provide an excellent opportunity for the musical development and socialization of older adults. The advantage of using music ensembles for socialization purposes is that music is inherently nonthreatening and an inviting medium. Ensembles require camaraderie and a good working relationship among members. Another objective that can be achieved through these performing groups is the enhancement of memory skills. Learning and memorizing new music is an enjoyable and excellent strategy for exercising memory and other cognitive functions.

Special ensembles for older adults, such as those sponsored by New Horizons Music programs, have become widespread over the last two decades. The first New Horizons program, at the Eastman School of Music in Rochester, New York, was specifically designed to serve seniors 50 and over—the age of eligibility for joining the American Association of Retired Persons (AARP). New Horizons Music programs provide opportunities for adults to make music, including those who have had no musical training as well as those who have studied in school music programs but have been inactive since that time. The organizers' belief was that every person has musical potential that can be developed to a level that will be personally rewarding; hence, musical groups should be inclusive rather than exclusive. Unfortunately, many adults have been made to feel unmusical by parents or music teachers, and New Horizons Music programs have done much to reeducate older adults about their musical potential. The concept and philosophy of New Horizons Music programs can be applied to many other types of music making and music classes. Learning music with others, as students do in school, is fun, and many older adults have discovered that joy. Intergenerational music groups of older adults and students provide an added dimension of diversity and foster understanding and acceptance of both age groups (Darrow, Johnson, & Ollenberger, 1994). Music learning and music making with others can provide a sense of personal well-being, which is often lacking in many aging adults.

PSYCHOSOCIAL WELL-BEING

Older adults often experience negative emotions and feelings of isolation that can keep them from optimal levels of wellness. They often lack a support system and a sense of connection to others, and they can feel isolated from the community around them. These emotional needs can be met by promoting older persons' participation in group music therapy activities. These activities can help them build relationships and have positive experiences with others, which can ultimately lead to increased opportunities for socialization. Participation in group music therapy activities can also elevate older persons' mood and, consequently, increase their energy level. Older adults can also participate in performing groups such as church or community choirs, senior adult bands, or drumming circles. Such musical groups can provide seniors, who are often removed from their families, with a support system, companionship, and a sense of connection to others. Other types of music therapy activities can also assist in meeting their emotional needs and can work toward achieving a sense of overall well-being. Increased self-esteem and decreased symptoms of depression both contribute to one's well-being.

The Use of Music to Increase Self-Esteem

- Music therapy interventions such as lyric analysis can help older adults identify and express current feelings about their self-worth and their environment.
- Songwriting activities can provide older adults an outlet for expression and a nonthreatening forum for sharing feelings. The songwriting product can instill in the older adult a sense of pride and productivity. Songs can also be recorded to share with family and friends to increase positive socialization with others.
- Participation in group music therapy activities can assist older adults in building relationships and having positive experiences with others, which can lead to increased self-esteem.

The Use of Music to Decrease Symptoms of Depression

- One-to-one sessions of active music making with a music therapist can build rapport and trust and can provide an opportunity for sharing.
- Music therapy interventions, such as lyric analysis, can be used to help older adults identify feelings in a song that may be similar to their own or to identify lyrics that express the cause(s) of their depression; however, lyrics can also be used to verbalize individuals' hopes for the future.
- Group music therapy activities can elevate participants' mood and increase their energy level, particularly those activities that also have a physical component, such as moving or dancing to music. Dancing provides opportunities for socialization and support building that can lead to reduced stress.

Stress management is an important component of wellness programs for older adults. Proper stress management can lead to an improved emotional state, more restful sleep, and increased energy. Music therapists can teach older adults to identify stressors and stress responses. Then, once stressors are identified, music therapists can teach seniors how to use music to relieve stress symptoms, such as singing or deep breathing to music, and how to employ these stress-relieving techniques at home.

Finally, for older adults who have trouble falling asleep or staying asleep, music therapists can employ music techniques to address sleep habits. The music therapist can create a CD with patient-preferred music designed to help the client structure and facilitate the act of falling asleep. Use of the selected music can be used as a cue that it is time to sleep, thus improving restfulness and possibly decreasing stress. Many of the interventions discussed in prior chapters are also applicable to wellness, such as strategies for reducing stress and promoting relaxation.

COGNITIVE STIMULATION

Cognitive stimulation and physical conditioning are two of the most essential components of wellness programs for older adults. Maintaining mental and physical well-being are key concerns of individuals as they age. Cognitive stimulation consists of planned interventions designed to promote mental awareness and comprehension. Such interventions are particularly important for older adults, as cognitive decline is one of the common characteristics associated with aging. Cognition is complex and is a combination of various mental skills (Park, 1992).

Cognition is a combination of skills, including

- attention
- learning
- memory
- language and speech
- fine motor skills
- visuospatial orientation
- executive functions, such as goal-setting, planning, and judgment

Most cognitive processes decline with age, though some are more affected than others. These processes have all shown age effects:

- processes involving attention
- working memory capabilities (the amount of information processed without losing track of any information)
- understanding written text
- making inferences
- encoding (putting information into memory) and retrieval (retrieving information from memory) (Park, 1992, p. 453)

Other processes show little or no decline with age, such as

- picture recognition
- implicit memory (information that is unconscientiously remembered, such as a fear response)
- prospective memory (remembering to watch favorite TV program)

Additionally, older adults' performance on highly practiced expert skills can equal those of young adults (e.g., playing an instrument, typing, playing bridge or chess). There is considerable variation in cognitive decline among individuals, and cognitive decline is not inevitable. Many fortunate older adults appear to avoid cognitive decline. Some risk factors for cognitive decline are potentially manageable.

Music therapy can serve as a useful management strategy for individuals at all levels of cognitive decline and with varying types of decline. The three major types of cognitive decline associated with aging are

1. Age-Associated Memory Impairment (AAMI)—mild memory impairment that can occur with normal aging but cannot be detected with objective psychometric testing for the person's age group

2. Mild Cognitive Impairment (MCI)—mild memory loss that can be detected with objective psychometric testing for the person's age group

3. Dementia (includes Alzheimer's disease)—chronic, progressive, irreversible, global cognitive impairment and memory loss that are severe enough to affect daily functioning (Park, 1992)

For individuals with mild declines or those associated with typical aging, music can be used to enhance the recall of information. Remembering the sequential order of the 26 letters of the alphabet is one example of music as a mnemonic device. Lyric analysis or composing songs is one music strategy used to practice written and verbal language skills. Composing and performing music, or researching and learning about music, are also enjoyable ways to keep the mind active. For individuals with advanced cognitive declines, music can provide comfort and familiarity, reduce agitation and apathy, afford opportunities for nonthreatening socialization, and promote caregiver bonding (Gallagher, Lagman, Walsh, Davis, & LeGrand, 2006; Giaquinto, Cacciato, Minasi, Sostero, & Amanda, 2006; Raglio et al., 2008; Thompson, Moulin, Hayre, & Jones, 2005; Ziv, Granot, Hai, Dassa, & Haimov, 2007).

Music therapists and researchers have employed numerous interventions with persons who are in varied stages of cognitive decline. Researchers have been primarily concerned with maintaining communicative skills, increasing active participation and social behaviors, and improving language functioning (Brotons & Pickett-Cooper, 1996; Cevasco & Grant, 2003; Clair & Bernstein, 1990; Clair, Mathews, & Kosloski, 2005; Hanson, Gfeller, Woodworth, Swanson, & Garand, 1996; Olderog-Millard & Smith, 1989; Pollack & Namazi, 1992). Other cognitive stimulation objectives and evidenced-based outcomes are to

1. stimulate long-term memory (Wylie, 1990);

2. improve short-term memory and other cognitive abilities (reduce confusion, improve retention of information, enhance category fluency, etc.) (Bruer, Spitznagel, & Cloninger, 2007; Gregory, 2002; Groene, 2001; Prickett & Moore, 1991; Reigler, 1980; Thompson et al., 2005; Van de Winckel, Feys, De Weerdt, & Dom, 2004);

3. improve reality orientation (Smith-Marchese, 1994);

4. improve verbal skills (Brotons & Koger, 2000);

5. enhance reminiscence (Byrne, 1982; Wylie, 1990);

6. assist in recalling information (Aldridge & Aldridge, 1992; Depperschmidt, 1992; Foster & Valentine, 2001; Lipe, 1995; Prickett & Moore, 1991; Sambandham & Schirm, 1995).

CONCLUSION

Music therapy offers a unique component to the field of health and wellness. Listening to music and creating music, alone or with others, can be incorporated into nearly every area of wellness. Music therapists can design music activities for older adults in groups or in one-to-one sessions to meet specific goals directed toward increasing holistic wellness and improving overall quality of life. Music therapy interventions overlap into several areas of wellness (physical, emotional, social); thus, increasing wellness in one area often leads to an increase in another area. The greatest attribute of music participation is its availability and accessibility to any individual who has an interest. Research in music and wellness lends support to the benefits of music interventions in nearly all facets of wellness.

REFERENCES

Administration on Aging. (2008). *Aging statistics*. Washington, DC: Author.

Aldridge, D., & Aldridge, G. (1992). Two epistemologies: Music therapy and medicine in the treatment of dementia. *The Arts in Psychotherapy, 19*, 243–255.

American Music Therapy Association (AMTA). (2005). *AMTA Standards of Clinical Practice*. Silver Spring, MD: Author.

Benson, E. R., & McDevitt, J. Q. (1989). Home care and the older adult: Illness care versus wellness care. *Holistic Nursing Practice, 3*(2), 30–38.

Bittman, B., Berk, L., Shannon, M., Sharaf, M., Westengard, J., Guegler, K. J., & Ruff, D. W. (2005). Recreational music-making modulates the human stress response: A preliminary individualized gene expression strategy. *Medical Science Monitor, 11*(2), BR31–BR40.

Brotons, M., & Koger, S. (2000). The impact of music therapy on language functioning in dementia. *Journal of Music Therapy, 37*, 183–195.

Brotons, M., & Pickett-Cooper, P. (1996). The effects of music therapy intervention on agitation behaviors of Alzheimer's disease patients. *Journal of Music Therapy, 33*, 2–18.

Bruer, A. B., Spitznagel, E., & Cloninger, C. R. (2007). The temporal limits of cognitive change from music therapy in elderly persons with dementia or dementia-like cognitive impairment: A randomized controlled trial. *Journal of Music Therapy, 44*(4), 308–328.

Bugos, J. A. (2007). Individualized piano instruction enhances executive functioning and working memory in older adults. *Aging and Mental Health, 11*(4), 464–471.

Byrne, L. A. (1982). Music therapy and reminiscence: A case study. *Clinical Gerontologist, 1*, 76–77.

Cevasco, A. M., & Grant, R. E. (2003). Comparisons for different methods for eliciting exercise-to-music for clients with Alzheimer's disease. *Journal of Music Therapy, 40*, 41–56.

Clair, A. A., & Bernstein, B. (1990). A comparison of singing, vibrotactile and nonvibrotactile instrumental playing responses in severely regressed persons with dementia of the Alzheimer's type. *Journal of Music Therapy, 27*, 119–125.

Clair, A. A., Mathews, R. M., & Kosloski, K. (2005). Assessment of active music participation as an indication of subsequent music making engagement for persons with midstage dementia. *American Journal of Alzheimer's Disease and Other Dementias, 20*(1), 37–40.

Clair, A. A., & Memmott, J. (2008). *Therapeutic uses of music with older adults*. Silver Spring, MD: American Music Therapy Association.

Darrow, A. A., Johnson, C. M., & Ollenberger, T. (1994). The effect of participation in an intergenerational choir on teens' and older persons' cross-age attitudes. *Journal of Music Therapy, 31*, 119–134.

Depperschmidt, K. A. (1992). *Musical mnemonics as an aid to memory in patients with dementia of the Alzheimer's type.* Unpublished master's thesis, Colorado State University, Ft. Collins.

Foster, N. A., & Valentine, E. R. (2001). The effect of auditory stimulation on auto-biographical recall in dementia. *Experimental Aging Research, 27*, 215–228.

Gallagher, L. M., Lagman, R., Walsh, D., Davis, M. P., & LeGrand, S. B. (2006). The clinical effects of music therapy in palliative medicine. *Supportive Care in Cancer, 14*, 859–866.

Ghetti, C. M., Hama, M., Woolrich, J. (2008). Wellness and music therapy. In A. A. Darrow (Ed.), *Introduction to approaches in music therapy* (2nd ed., pp. 131–151). Silver Spring, MD: American Music Therapy Association.

Giaquinto, S., Cacciato, A., Minasi, S., Sostero, E., & Amanda, S. (2006). Effects of music-based therapy on distress following knee arthroplasty. *British Journal of Nursing, 15*(10), 576–579.

Gibbons, A. C. (1983). Primary measures of music audiation scores in an institutionalized elderly population. *Journal of Music Therapy, 20*, 21–29.

Grape, C., Sandgren, M., Hansson, L. O., Ericson, M., & Theorell T. (2003). Does singing promote well-being? An empirical study of professional and amateur singers during a singing lesson. *Integrative Physiological and Behavioral Science, 38*, 65–74.

Gregory, D. (2002). Music listening for maintaining attention of older adults with cognitive impairments. *Journal of Music Therapy, 39,* 244–264.

Groene, R. W. (2001). The effect of presentation and accompaniment style on attentional and responsive behaviors of participants with dementia diagnoses. *Journal of Music Therapy, 38*, 36–50.

Gutt, C. A. (1996). Health and wellness in the community. In J. M. Cookfair (Ed.), *Nursing care in the community* (2nd ed., pp. 143–174). St. Louis, MO: Mosby.

Hamburg, J., & Clair, A. A. (2003). The effects of a movement with music program on measures of balance and gait speed in healthy older adults. *Journal of Music Therapy, 40*(3), 212–226.

Hanser, S. B. (1990). A music therapy strategy for depressed older adults in the community. *Journal of Applied Gerontology, 9*, 283–298.

Hanser, S. B., & Thompson, L. W. (1994). Effects of a music therapy strategy on depressed older adults. *Journal of Gerontology, 49*(6), 265–269.

Hanson, N., Gfeller, K., Woodworth, G., Swanson, E. A., & Garand, L. (1996). A comparison of the effectiveness of differing types and difficulty of music activities in programming for older adults with Alzheimer's disease and related disorders. *Journal of Music Therapy, 33*, 93–123.

Johnson, G., Otto, D., & Clair, A. A. (2001). The effect of instrumental and vocal music on the adherence to a physical rehabilitation exercise program with persons who are elderly. *Journal of Music Therapy, 38*, 82–96.

Johnson, J. E. (2003). The use of music to promote sleep in older women. *Journal of Community Health Nursing, 20*(1), 27–35.

Lai, H. L., & Good, M. (2005). Music improves sleep quality in older adults. *Journal of Advanced Nursing, 49*(3), 234–244.

Lipe, A. (1995). The use of music performance tasks in the assessment of cognitive functioning among older adults with dementia. *Journal of Music Therapy, 32*, 137–151.

Mornhinweg, G. C., & Voignier, R. R. (1995). Music for sleep disturbance in the elderly. *Journal of Holistic Nursing, 13*(3), 248–254.

Olderog-Millard, K. A., & Smith, J. M. (1989). The influence of group singing therapy on the behavior of Alzheimer's disease patients. *Journal of Music Therapy, 5*, 58–70.

Park, D. C. (1992). Applied cognitive aging research. In F. I. M. Craik & T. A. Salthouse (Eds.), *The handbook of aging and cognition* (pp. 449–493). Hillsdale, NJ: Lawrence Erlbaum Associates.

Pelletier, C. L. (2004). The effect of music on decreasing arousal due to stress: A meta-analysis. *Journal of Music Therapy, 41*, 192–214.

Pollock, N., & Namazi, K. (1992). The effect of music participation on the social behavior of Alzheimer's patients. *Journal of Music Therapy, 29*, 54–67.

Prickett, C. A., & Moore, R. S. (1991). The effects of music to aid memory of Alzheimer's patients. *Journal of Music Therapy, 28*, 102–110.

Raglio, A., Bellelli, G., Traficante, D., Gianotti, M., Ubezio, M. C., Villani, D., & Trabucchi, M. (2008). Efficacy of music therapy in the treatment of behavioral and psychiatric symptoms of dementia. *Alzheimer Disease & Associated Disorders, 22*, 158–162.

Reigler, J. (1980). Comparison of a reality orientation program for geriatric patients with and without music. *Journal of Music Therapy, 17*, 26–33.

Sambandham, M., & Schirm, V. (1995). Music as a nursing intervention for residents with Alzheimer's disease in long-term care. *Geriatric Nursing, 16*, 79–83.

Smith-Marchese, K. (1994). The effects of participatory music on the reality orientation and sociability of Alzheimer's residents in a long-term-care setting. *Activities, Adaptation, and Aging, 18*(2), 41–55.

Thompson, R. G., Moulin, C. J. A., Hayre, S., & Jones, R. W. (2005). Music enhances category fluency in healthy older adults and Alzheimer's disease patients. *Experimental Aging Research, 31*(1), 91–99.

Van de Winckel, A., Feys, H., De Weerdt, W., & Dom, R. (2004). Cognitive and behavioral effects of music-based exercises in patients with dementia. *Clinical Rehabilitation, 18*(3), 253–260.

Walker, S. N. (1991). Wellness and aging. In E. M. Baines (Ed.), *Perspectives on gerontological nursing* (pp. 41–58). Newbury Park, CA: Sage.

Wylie, M. E. (1990). A comparison of the effects of old familiar songs, antique objects, historical summaries, and general questions on the reminiscence of nursing-home residents. *Journal of Music Therapy, 27*, 2–12.

Zelazny, C. M. (2001). Therapeutic instrumental music playing in hand rehabilitation for older adults with osteoarthritis: Four case studies. *Journal of Music Therapy, 38*, 97–113.

Ziv, N., Granot, A., Hai, S., Dassa, A., & Haimov, I. (2007). The effect of background stimulative music on behavior in Alzheimer's patients. *Journal of Music Therapy, 44*(4), 329–343.

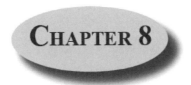

CHAPTER 8

REVIEW OF THE RESEARCH LITERATURE ON WELLNESS AND MUSIC THERAPY

Increased awareness regarding the importance of a healthy lifestyle has resulted in more seniors actively engaging in behaviors conducive to good health. Much of the public awareness has been a result of recent research annotated in news releases and popular press—AARP publications in particular. The original research, published mainly in aging and healthcare journals, has shown the effects of exercise, nutrition, socialization, and other components of wellness programs on the quality of life and health of older adults (Miller, 1991). Some researchers have conjectured that because many music therapy activities require social engagement, they may be more appealing to older adults than other types of wellness activities, and thus increase adherence to long-term lifestyle changes (VanWeelden & Whipple, 2004). Clair and Memmott (2008) have also identified the aptness of music therapy to achieve wellness goals and, consequently, as the baby boomer generation ages, they foresee an increased demand for research that results in evidence-based practice.

The past decade has brought a substantial increase in research evaluating the impact of wellness programs on the health of older adults. The demand for evidence-based practice has moved beyond the medical field to therapeutic interventions, including music therapy. The impetus for evidence-based practice was a result of insurance providers' request to secure data that indicated medical and therapeutic interventions were effective, before approving funding for treatment (Shapiro, Lasker, Bindman, & Lee, 1993). As a result, researchers have attempted to respond with empirical evidence that substantiates the clinical outcomes of various medical treatments and therapeutic interventions.

For many years, the effectiveness of wellness programs was supported mostly by anecdotal assertions. Over the past 20 years, however, researchers have provided evidence to substantiate claims of their effectiveness (Jensen & Allen, 1994). The evidence suggests that wellness programs have positive effects on consumer outcomes. There is a perception of efficacy among consumers who participate in wellness programs, as well as the suggestion that participation reduces the need for more costly health services. There is also a suggestion that this type of intervention reduces health service usage (Watt, Verma, & Flynn, 1998). Research has shown that older adults' functional abilities, general state of wellness, and perceived quality of life are all important factors in the success of medical interventions and in patients' adherence to treatment regimens (Clair, 2008). Personal wellness and its influence on the physicians' choice of medical treatments demonstrate the complexities of evidence-based medicine and, subsequently, the need for collaboration across disciplines to facilitate the best patient outcomes (Daly, 2005). Music therapists seeking reimbursement for services have become acutely aware of the need to produce evidence for treatment outcomes. The provision of measurable, evidence-based outcomes in music therapy remains a top priority as music therapists work to ensure optimum quality of life for older adults.

RESEARCH IN MUSIC THERAPY AND WELLNESS

Music is currently being employed in a variety of ways that address various dimensions of wellness in older adults—with the primary dimensions being physical fitness, psychosocial well-being, and cognitive stimulation (Koga & Tims, 2001). Researchers have found that music provides meaning to people's lives, and that its mere presence often contributes to a general sense of well-being (Hays, 2006). Hays, Bright, and Minichiello (2002) found that many people value music and consider it to be an important part of their everyday lives, though the purposes of its use are varied: recreational, educational, social, emotional, therapeutic, and spiritual.

In related later studies, researchers examined the importance of music in facilitating well-being and music's contribution to older adults' quality of life (Laukka, 2007). The data derived from qualitative interviews revealed that music provides many adults with ways of feeling competent, less isolated, and connected with other people, and with a greater sense of good health. Hays (2006) concluded that music facilitates meaning in people's lives and that it is associated with the quality of their emotional and life experiences. Laukka (2007) also found that listening to music is a frequent source of positive emotions for older adults. Participants reported using music listening for pleasure, mood regulation, and relaxation. Although health status and personality were found to be the most important predictors of well-being, some listening strategies were also significantly related to psychological well-being. The results give important insights into older adults' uses of music in everyday life and possible relationships between musical activities and well-being.

One of the earliest studies addressing the importance of music to older adults was also one of the few experimental studies found (VanderArk, Newman, & Bell, 1983). Residents in two nursing homes were matched on age-related variables. Residents in one nursing home had music for 45 minutes twice a week for 5 weeks. During music sessions, residents sang and played instruments to familiar songs. When compared to residents in the nursing home without music, those receiving music had significantly higher ratings of life satisfaction, attitudes toward music, and music self-concept.

Beyond the purposes of music for life meaning and general well-being, a number of researchers have been concerned with the effect of music activities, both active and passive, on various states of wellness. Researchers have examined the effects of music interventions on older adults' physical functioning, health-related behaviors, and psychosocial well-being. Related to these areas of health, research with older adults has shown that music therapy interventions can

1. increase motivation and compliance with physical exercise (Cevasco & Grant, 2003; Johnson, Otto, & Clair, 2001);
2. provide opportunities for meaningful interaction with peers to reduce isolation (Coffman, 2002; Coffman & Adamek, 1999; Darrow, Johnson, & Ollenberger, 1994);
3. provide an outlet for emotional expression to reduce anxiety and stress (Raglio et al., 2008; Suzuki, Kanamori, Nagasawa, Tokiko, & Takayoki, 2007); and
4. stimulate active cognitive functioning (Foster & Valentine, 2001; Gregory, 2002).

Older adults need not be musical in order to participate in music therapy activities. Music interventions can be tailored to clients' past experiences with music, as well as to their musical style and medium preferences. Gibbons (1988) found that older adults generally prefer music that was popular during their teen and young adult years; however, recent research indicates that seniors can also enjoy learning new music—music that was popular during their children's young adult years, and even music popular with their grandchildren (Belgrave & Darrow, 2007). Researchers have examined the effectiveness of various musical interventions used with older adults and found that singing is generally thought to be the most accessible music medium for older adults; however, research indicates that a variety of musical interventions can be effective with seniors:

1. singing (Bowers, 1998; Grape, Sandgren, Hansson, Ericson, & Theorell; 2003)
2. playing music (Clair, 1998; Coffman & Adamek, 1999)
3. therapeutic drumming (Bittman et al., 2001)
4. music listening (Batt-Rawden, 2006; Sloboda & O'Neill, 2001)
5. music-assisted movement programs (Hamburg & Clair, 2003, 2004)
6. guided imagery and music (McKinney, Antoni, Kumar, Tims, & McCabe, 1997)
7. lyric analysis (O'Callaghan & Grocke, 2009).

These various music interventions provide a constructive approach to wellness for older adults because researchers have found that most adults have musical abilities, and unlike many cognitive and physical abilities, musicality does not decrease with age (Gibbons, 1982a, 1982b, 1983). The longevity of musical ability adds to its viability as a therapeutic agent. With the numerous rehabilitation and senior living facilities offering music programs to their residents, music therapists are finding increased employment in wellness programs each year (AMTA, 2009; Smith & Lipe, 1991).

RESEARCH IN MUSIC AND PHYSICAL WELL-BEING

Music as an Accompaniment to Exercise

Regular exercise promotes health and well-being in older adults through increased physical flexibility and strength, improved balance, mood, and cognition (Clair & Memmott, 2008). Exercise also protects against age-related complications such as heart disease, cholesterol, and high blood pressure. Most traditional exercise classes incorporate some type of background music. Music has been found to increase the enjoyment of exercise, enhance older adults' motivation to exercise, and structure exercise movements (Weideman, 1986). Enjoyment, motivation, and structure all contribute to the benefits of exercise for older adults (Clair, 1996).

There are musical elements that also contribute to the benefits of exercise as well as to older adults' commitment to an exercise regime. The selection of music is generally based on the music's tempo and style. Tempo is the most important musical element associated with exercise (Wininger & Pargman, 2003). In order to strengthen older adults' exercise compliance, the tempo of music should be matched to an individual's functional abilities and to the purpose of the exercise. Hamburg and Clair's research (2003, 2004) suggests that other aspects of rhythm are also important. They found that the rhythmic durations of music influence the length and range of individuals' physical movements. Various researchers have found that the use of music during exercise results in higher recovery of heart rates, longer periods of exercise, greater breath capacity, general physical function, and commitment to exercise (Beckett, 1990; Hagen, Armstrong-Esther, & Sandilands, 2003; Johnson et al., 2001; McBride, Graydon, Sidani, & Hall, 1999).

In a study by Teel, Carson, Hamburg, and Clair (1999), a 20-minute program of 14 movement sequences set to music was developed and offered to older adults. The program did not incorporate traditional exercises but rather creative movements sequenced to the music. Participants learned new movements during the first 5 weeks and reviewed all movement sequences the 6th week. Participants reported benefits of the program such as enhanced posture awareness, improved sense of balance, and increased social interactions. The movement program utilized music unfamiliar to the participants. Researchers suggested that, in future research, the use of familiar music may influence participants' practice outside the sessions.

Popular or preferred music is often used to accompany exercises (Hagen et al., 2003); however, Hamburg and Clair (2003) examined the effect of instrumental music specifically composed to indicate movement formations for an exercise program targeted at older adults. They found that participants' weekly participation in the wellness-based movement and music program led to increases in one-foot stance balance, gait speed, and functional reach after five sessions. In a later larger study, their findings were corroborated when participants also demonstrated improved measures of balance and gait after their participation in the music and movement protocol (Hamburg & Clair, 2004). In their physical rehabilitation exercise program, Johnson et al. (2001) found that vocal music, as well as instrumental music, is effective with older adults, and that both are preferred to no music during exercise.

Improvements in physical functioning are often related to associated gains in cognitive functioning. In a study designed to compare music exercise and traditional occupational therapy (OT) activities and their effects on physical and cognitive functioning, music exercise was shown to result in significant improvements in more areas than OT alone, though both types of therapy were associated with physical and cognitive gains (Hagen et al., 2003). Such music exercise programs have the potential to promote gains in older adults' physical functioning and thus assist in maintaining independence and improving quality of life. Older adults who exercise to music may find that music is a distracter to the discomfort they experience when executing strenuous exercises. Past research has shown music's ability to mask the perception of pain (Mitchell & McDonald, 2006).

Music and Management of Pain

Most individuals experience some type of pain due to the effects of aging. Osteoarthritis and accompanying joint pain is the most common type of physical pain experienced by older adults. Osteoarthritis is a group of diseases and mechanical abnormalities involving degradation of joints, and it is the most common degenerative disease among older adults. It usually begins in middle age and is progressive throughout the lifespan. Chronic pain associated with osteoarthritis can be an obstacle in maintaining daily living activities and physical independence.

Researchers have examined the effect of music on reducing the perception of osteoarthritis pain experienced by older adults and have found that music listening is a useful distracter to pain (McCaffrey & Freeman, 2003; Siedliecki & Good, 2006; Zelazny, 2001). In Siedliecki and Good's (2006) study, participants with continuous pain in two or more body parts listened to music on headsets for an hour a day with half choosing the music they listened to and half choosing from relaxation recordings provided to them. A control group did not listen to any music. Findings revealed a significant decrease in pain levels with music therapy and no significant difference between participants who chose their own music and those who selected music from the selected list. In another study utilizing music listening as the intervention (McCaffrey & Freeman, 2003), older adults listened to music for 20 minutes per day and were compared to control participants who sat quietly for 20 minutes per day. The researchers found that participants who listened to music reported significantly less pain than those who sat quietly, concluding that music listening is an effective intervention for older adults experiencing chronic pain due to osteoarthritis.

Music listening is a passive activity. To investigate the effect of more active music making on the perception of osteoarthritis pain, Zelazny (2001) examined the effects of keyboard playing on the management of hand osteoarthritis in older adults. Four participants, with diagnoses of hand osteoarthritis, met the investigator 4 days a week, for approximately 30 minutes, for 4 weeks. Participants played folk and big band melodies on a Yamaha PSR-510 touch-sensitive electronic keyboard for 20 minutes each session. Evaluation included pre- and post-study occupational therapy measures of finger pinch meter and range of motion. Participants assessed arthritic discomfort using a visual Likert scale (1–10) before and after each session. A MIDI sequencing computer program, Master Tracks Pro, measured finger velocity, before and after each session. Results indicated that finger pinch meter readings and range of motion were positively increased by keyboard playing. Two participants recorded significant decreases in arthritic discomfort after playing, while three participants showed significant improvement in finger velocity and, hence, finger strength/dexterity due to treatment. Participants enjoyed the treatments, with additional benefits being improved structure of leisure time and increased socialization with other adults. Older adults with osteoarthritis often isolate themselves due to the disabling effects of the disease.

Researchers have also examined the use of music to reduce older adults' perception of pain after undergoing hip and knee surgery, and in the management of chronic osteoarthritis (Buchhaupt, 2000; McCaffrey & Locsin, 2006; Siedliecki & Good, 2006). McCaffrey and Locsin (2006) examined the effects of music listening with older adults following hip and knee surgery and found a reduction in confusion and pain, improved ambulation, and higher satisfaction scores in those who listened to music. These findings have strong implications for practice, since pain and acute confusion after surgery can increase patients' hospital stay and reduce their physical functioning. Additionally, music listening to relieve pain perception is a strategy that can be carried out by nursing staff as well as music therapists.

Chronic pain frequently results in secondary conditions such as stress and anxiety. It may also contribute to decreased physical activity due to an individual's apprehension of exacerbating pain. Inactivity, in turn, leads to greater pain when the older adult ultimately attempts to engage in physical activities. Music has been shown not only to be a distracter to pain (Mitchell & MacDonald, 2006) but also to reduce the stress associated with pain (Pelletier, 2004) and with other age-related conditions such as chronic heart disease (Bradt & Dileo, 2009), pulmonary disorders (McBride et al., 1999), and depression (Hanser & Thompson, 1994). Studies demonstrating the ability of music to mask pain are important beyond participants' reduced perception of pain. If left untreated, chronic pain can lead to severe emotional symptoms in older adults. There is a strong relationship between chronic pain and stress among older adults.

Use of Music to Reduce Stress

Researchers suggest that the rhythm of music can have a calming effect on most individuals, but particularly on those experiencing stress due to pain (McBride et al., 1999; Pelletier, 2004). In a meta-analysis of studies examining the effect of music on stress, Pelletier (2004) found that stress reduction was significantly different depending on participants' age, the type of stress experienced, and the type of intervention employed. Several studies have shown that older adults with the following diagnoses have experienced a reduction in stress and anxiety as a result of music listening interventions:

- cardiovascular surgery—less stress by listening to music (Twiss, Seaver, & McCaffrey, 2006)
- chronic obstructive pulmonary disease (COPD)—less anxiety by listening to preferred music (McBride et al., 1999)
- coronary heart disease—less stress and anxiety by listening to music (Bradt & Dileo, 2009)
- age-related depression—less stress by listening to music for relaxation, reflection, guided reminiscence, and change of mood state (Hanser & Thompson, 1994; Maratos, Gold, Wang, & Crawford, 2008).

Other researchers have found that adults experienced an elevation in mood and reduced levels of hormones associated with stress by participating in guided imagery and music (GIM) (McKinney et al., 1997). These findings indicate that music listening, with or without imagery, is an effective intervention for relieving stress that is due to a variety of both physical and emotional etiologies.

Depression is a frequent outcome of stress, though the relationship between stress and depression is more complex. Frequent periods of stress may result in depression; however, stress can also be exacerbated by chronic depression. Studies have indicated that nearly half of all nursing home residents experience depression (Harris, 2007). Older adults do not experience the same kind of stress factors they experienced earlier in their life (career demands, child rearing); however, they frequently experience depression due to other factors such as the loss of a spouse, declining health, and greater physical dependency. Eight to 20% of older adults in the community suffer from depressive symptoms (U.S. Public Health Service, 2009).

Because depression is common in the aging population (Sadovsky, 1998), researchers examined a music therapy strategy for relieving symptoms of depression in older adults (Hanser, 1990; Hanser & Thompson, 1994). Hanser's (1990) music therapy strategy for depressed older adults involved eight music-listening programs for home use. The strategy utilized body relaxation, imagery, stimulation, and sleep enhancement with music to cue relaxation and positive thinking. Participants with major or minor depressive disorders demonstrated positive gains on several depression inventories after participating in the 8-week program. The music therapy program demonstrated potential as a low-cost, home-based treatment for depressed older adults. The effectiveness of the music therapy program was further substantiated by comparing participants who were involved in a music therapist-administered program, a self-administered program, or a wait-list control group. Participants in both music conditions performed significantly better than the control participants on standardized tests of depression, distress, self-esteem, and mood. These improvements were clinically significant and were maintained over a 9-month follow-up period (Hanser & Thompson, 1994).

These aforementioned studies indicate that music listening is a viable intervention for reducing indicators of stress and depression in older adults. In a meta-analysis of music and stress studies, participants' music preferences were a possible factor in the effectiveness of music listening to reduce stress and anxiety (Pelletier, 2004).

Use of Music to Address Other Age-Related Physical Conditions

The careful selection of music for listening has also been shown to be a variable in the effectiveness of music with other types of age-related conditions such as tinnitus, emphysema, and hypertension. Tinnitus is characterized by annoying ringing, buzzing, whistling, hissing, or other noises in the ear. It primarily affects older adults, though it can be experienced by younger adults, especially those who have been exposed to loud, amplified music or other extreme, sustained noises. Tinnitus can affect older adults' sleep, concentration, and mood. Music, as well as engineered environmental sounds such as rain or ocean waves, is often used to mask tinnitus. However, in a recent study, Okamoto, Stracke, Stoll, and Pantev (2009) found that it might be possible to actually reverse ringing in the ears by altering music to include frequencies other than those that cause the ringing. Rather than simply masking, the researchers attempted to reduce tinnitus loudness by having chronic tinnitus patients listen to their preferred music, which was modified ("notched") to contain no energy in the frequency range surrounding the individual tinnitus frequency. After 12 months of regular listening, the experimental group showed significantly reduced subjective tinnitus loudness and, more importantly, exhibited reduced evoked activity in auditory cortex areas corresponding to the tinnitus frequency compared to those in the control group, who had received the placebo notched music intervention. These findings indicate the potential to reverse maladaptive auditory cortex activity and indicate that tinnitus loudness can be significantly diminished by an enjoyable, low-cost intervention using tailored music.

Another age-related chronic condition that is debilitating for many older adults is emphysema, a long-term, progressive disease of the lung that causes shortness of breath. Research has shown that singing can help increase or maintain the level of respiratory function in individuals with emphysema (Engen, 2005). In Engen's (2005) study, seniors with emphysema who were non-singers participated in twelve 45-minute vocal classes in small groups. Warm-ups included blowing props such as pinwheels to control airflow. Also included in the intervention were group sing-alongs to reinforce concepts of deep breathing. A 2-week follow-up revealed that the seniors were continuing to use diaphragmatic breathing and reported a psychological benefit to the vocal classes.

Hypertension, commonly known as high blood pressure, is another condition often associated with aging. A risk factor for strokes and heart attacks, hypertension is the leading cause of renal failure and may also be a predictor of dementia (Pierdomenico et al., 2009). High blood pressure is common in older adults because blood vessels become less elastic and stiffen with age, thus restricting the flow of blood. Researchers found that individuals with mild hypertension who listened to classical, Celtic, or Indian (raga) music for just 30 minutes a day for 1 month had significant reductions in their blood pressure (Modesti et al., 2008). In contrast, participants in the control group, who made no changes in their daily routine, experienced only small, nonsignificant reductions in blood pressure. Another study revealed that listening to fast music increases blood pressure, whereas listening to slower music has the opposite effect (Bernardi, Porta, & Sleight, 2006). Randomly introducing pauses into the music lowers blood pressure even further. These effects are particularly marked in people who have had musical training. Other researchers have found that adults experienced a decrease in blood pressure by participating in music listening with guided imagery (McKinney et al., 1997). These data indicate that music listening may function as a nonpharmaceutical complementary treatment for hypertension.

USE OF MUSIC TO ADDRESS PSYCHOSOCIAL WELL-BEING

The effects of aging have the potential to affect all areas of psychosocial well-being: personal autonomy, environmental mastery, personal growth, self-perception, and relations with others. *Physical well-being* relates to one's ability to function normally in daily living activities such as bathing, dressing, eating, and mobility. *Mental well-being* assumes that one's cognitive faculties are intact and that there are no pressing concerns resulting in fear, anxiety, stress, depression, or other negative emotions. *Social well-being* implies one's ability to participate in society, to engage in interactions with others, and to fulfill roles as a family member, friend, worker, or community member (Frytak, 2000). As they age, many adults experience diminished capacities in one or more of these areas of psychosocial well-being. As reported in the previous sections of this chapter, music has the potential to address important aspects of physical well-being and mental well-being, as it relates to stress and depression. Aspects of older adults' social well-being can be addressed, in part, by encouraging their participation in lifelong learning programs. Lifelong learning can occur within any musical context; however, the structure provided by musical organizations such as community choirs and bands, or music classes offered at senior centers, is helpful in promoting learning.

Music and Lifelong Learning

Lifelong learning is the activity of participating in educational activities, seeking out new knowledge or developing a skill, formally or informally, over the course of a lifetime. Engaging in lifelong learning activities is especially important for older adults as it can assist in maintaining or augmenting physical, cognitive, and social functioning. As adults enter their later years, many experience the death of family members and friends, severely diminishing their social lives. Participating in music classes or activities can offer a new circle of friends and increased opportunities for socialization. A desire for socialization is the reason many older adults enroll in music activities, although many also have a strong desire to acquire or to improve music skills (Coffman, 2002; Coffman & Adamek, 2001). Learning or relearning music skills exercises active cognition and recall, employs fine motor skills, and promotes self-esteem and a sense of achievement (Ghetti, Hama, & Woolrich, 2008).

Various researchers have documented the importance of music in the lives of older adults and have suggested that music activities are easily accessible to most older adults because music is generally viewed a desirable activity and because it is adaptable to older adults' preferences and needs for adjustments in musical style, tempo, and loudness (Coffman, 2002; Cohen, Bailey, & Nilsson, 2002). Their data indicate that music is particularly effective as a social agent because most people enjoy music, and because music activities can be adapted for individuals with established music skills and for those with little to no musical background. Gibbons (1982b, 1983) found that older adults' abilities to acquire musical skills remain strong into their 90s, and that most older adults wish to advance their musical skills. In response to these research findings, various authors have developed music therapy programs for older adults (Douglass, 1985; Gibbons, 1984; Karras, 2001) and have written educational materials such as guitar or piano method books (Christiansen, 2007; Reuer, Crowe, & Bernstein, 2007). Some of these educational materials are specifically designed for the older adult, with large font and age-appropriate repertoire (Christiansen, 2007).

It may be that developing music skills is even more enjoyable and beneficial for individuals with little music training. Grape et al. (2003) found that amateur musicians reported joy and elatedness while participating in voice lessons. In addition, they felt more energetic and relaxed after the lessons. They also reported that they used the singing lessons as a means of self-actualization and self-expression and as a way to release emotional tension. The researchers concluded that singing lessons seemed to promote more well-being and less stress for amateurs when compared to professional singers.

Individuals who develop music skills through lessons are then able to participate in community musical groups. Participating in such groups provides the motivation to remain physically active and the opportunity to form new friendships. Older adults who participated in community music organizations, such as choirs and bands or music appreciation classes, reported enhanced quality of life and increased social relations (Coffman, 2002; Coffman & Adamek, 1999). Musical groups provide opportunities to form relationships with others who share similar interests and also reduce the possibility of isolation. The benefits of participating in musical organizations are not solely social, but also physical and cognitive. Group music lessons can stimulate cognitive activity as well as increase interpersonal interactions (Grape et al., 2003). Residents in a retirement village who participated in a facility chorus reported more satisfying social relations than those who did not participate (Wise, Hartmann, & Fisher, 1992). These data indicate that even informal vocal participation has the potential to promote overall wellness.

The purpose of a study by Cohen et al. (2006) was to measure the impact of professional music programs on the physical health, mental health, and social activities of adults 65 and older. Seniors averaging 80 years in age took part in choral programs at The Levine School of Music in Washington, D.C. After 2 years, when compared to a control group of similar individuals, the music participants

- reported better health and fewer falls;
- showed a slower rate of increase in doctor visits than nonparticipants;
- increased medication usage at a significantly lower rate than nonparticipants;
- showed greater improvements in depression, loneliness, and morale; and
- increased social interaction.

Though singing is generally considered to be the most accessible performance medium for older adults, playing piano is also accessible and is a skill highly valued among many older adults. Researchers have found that the development of piano skills need not be confined to youth—that older adults are fully capable of developing piano skills for personal enjoyment or as a leisure skill. Clair (1996) developed a wellness program for older adults that incorporated the use of piano keyboards. The wellness part of the program included breathing exercises, muscle relaxation exercises, cognitive strategies to encourage positive thinking and increase confidence, techniques for using music to stimulate or sedate behavior, and strategies for using music to influence mood. The wellness program was paired with weekly keyboard lessons. Decreases in anxiety, depression, and perception of loneliness were reported for individuals in the experimental group when compared to those in the control condition, who did not participate in the keyboard/wellness program (Bruhn & Clair, 1999; Koga & Tims, 2001).

Olsen (1984) was interested in the value of player piano music on the cognitive, behavioral, and affective responses of older adults. Eleven elderly clients in a retirement center participated in an ABA experimental design to measure responses to player piano music. Cognitive, affective, and behavioral data were collected through observational and subjective interview measures. Results demonstrated marked increases in physical responses to the musical intervention. Additionally, participants enjoyed player piano music, felt an enhanced state of well-being, and were able to retrieve specific long-term memories.

The Use of Music to Induce Relaxation and Sleep

Sleep is essential for health and well-being. It allows the body to rejuvenate and restore itself. Lack of sleep not only relates to chronic tiredness, but increases the risk of depression and anxiety and affects cognitive ability. Studies conclude that people who are sleep-deprived have significantly lower levels of performance in all areas compared to those who consistently sleep well (Banks & Dinger, 2007). Poor sleep is associated with a poorer quality of life. Unfortunately, older adults often experience problems with sleep. Researchers have found that older adults who have poor nighttime sleep are more likely to have depressed mood, attention and memory problems, excessive daytime sleepiness, and more nighttime falls (Kamel & Gammack, 2006). In a descriptive study, Mornhinweg and Voignier (1995) had participants who reported a sleep disturbance listen to classical and New Age music before bedtime. Participants kept daily sleep logs. Researchers found 96% of the participants reported improved sleep using the self-administered music intervention. These findings were corroborated in later larger studies that included additional factors related to healthy sleep. Music was shown to influence healthy sleep in older adults by reducing the time-to-sleep onset and the number of nighttime awakenings (Johnson, 2003). The findings of these two descriptive studies were strengthened by later research.

In a randomized control study by Lai and Good (2005), participants aged 60–83 years with difficulty in sleeping were recruited for study to examine the effect of music on sleep. Individuals reporting depression, cognitive impairment, medical or environmental problems that might interfere with sleep, and the use of sleeping medications or caffeine at bedtime were excluded. Participants listened to their choice of six 45-minute sedative music tapes at bedtime for 3 weeks. Music listening at bedtime resulted in significantly better sleep quality in the experimental group than in the control group, as well as significantly better components of sleep quality: better perceived sleep quality, longer sleep duration, greater sleep efficiency, shorter sleep latency, less sleep disturbance, and less daytime dysfunction.

Relaxation is a necessary precursor to sleep. It is also important in keeping stress levels down and in maintaining a functioning immune system. Music listening and music-regulated breathing exercises can assist in promoting both physical and mental relaxation (Krout, 2006; Lai, 2004). Krout (2006) offered information on the neurological bases of music listening, how music can be used in relaxation regimes, and factors to be considered when selecting music for relaxation. Lai (2004) investigated the importance of musical preferences as a factor in participants' relaxation responses to music. After determining participants' musical preferences, their heart rates and respiratory rates were measured before and after they listened to selected music. Participants were also asked to indicate the degree to which they liked the six types of soothing music. Results indicated participants' heart and respiratory rates were significantly lower after listening to music, and there were no differences among the types of music on relaxation. Researchers have suggested that music used for relaxation be sedative in nature, match the pace of the relaxation exercise, and be among the listener's musical preferences (Krout, 2006; Lai, 2004). The relaxation exercises used in music therapy wellness programs often include deep breathing, low stretching movements, and guided imagery techniques (Ghetti et al., 2008).

Music and Cognitive Stimulation in Older Adults

The maintenance of cognitive skills is important to the daily functioning of older adults. Hirokawa (2004) examined the effects of music listening and relaxation on arousal changes and the working memory of older adults. Fifteen female older adults participated in 10 minutes of three experimental conditions: (1) subject-preferred music, (2) relaxation instructions, and (3) silence control. Four subcategories of arousal—energy, tiredness, tension, and calmness—were measured before and after experimental treatment. After each experimental condition, participants completed a working memory task. Results indicated that music increased participants' energy levels, and relaxation and silence significantly decreased energy levels. All experimental conditions decreased subjects' tension levels. The scores on the working memory task were not significantly different among experimental conditions. Bugos (2007), however, found that piano instruction was a viable music intervention for stimulating working memory in older adults. In her study, neuropsychological assessments were administered at three time points: pre-training, following 6 months of intervention, and following a 3-month delay. The experimental group improved significantly on working memory measures compared to the control group. The results suggest that individualized piano instruction may be an effective intervention for some types of age-related cognitive decline.

Short-term memory is at particular risk for decline as one ages. A frequent complaint by older adults is an inability to recall names. Stull (2005) addressed this concern in her research by examining the effects of familiar music, unfamiliar music, and no music on face-name recall in aging adults. Participants in treatments 1 and 2 heard names set to either familiar music or unfamiliar music while they viewed the corresponding faces. Participants were invited to sing along as the song was sung three times. Participants in the control group condition heard the names spoken while they viewed the corresponding faces. Participants were then asked to recall as many names as possible (free recall); given a name, select the correct face from a closed response set of three faces (recognition); and recall the correct name for each face (face-name recall). Results indicated that differences in name recall were not significant; however, groups using music recalled more names than did the control group, and participants in the group using familiar music recalled more names than those in the group using unfamiliar music. These findings may have implications for daily use. Older adults who wish to recall names might find it helpful to associate song titles with a person's face. Possible song examples for women are "Goodnight Irene," "Once in Love with Amy," "K-K-K-Katy," "Annie's Song," "Barbara Ann," "Eleanor Rigby," "Georgia on My Mind," and "Peggy Sue." Possible song examples for men include "Danny Boy," "Tom Dooley," "Ben," "Brian's Song," "Johnny Be Good," "Frankie and Johnny," "Hit the Road, Jack," and "Big Bad John."

Cognitive skills can also be addressed not only by therapeutic interventions, but by engaging in music leisure activities. One longitudinal study revealed that older adults who regularly engaged in activities such as playing instruments, singing, and music-accompanied movement activities reduced their risk of Alzheimer's disease and other types of dementia. Researchers conjectured that such activities, which require the learning of new skills and are naturally reinforcing, prompt steady engagement and thus maintain important neurological activity (Verghese et al., 2003).

In a review of studies in which researchers investigated the independent and combined influences of age and experience on an assortment of long- and short-term musical memory tasks, Halpern (2002) found no simple relationship of aging to music cognition skills. Similar to Gibbons' (1982a, 1982b) findings, Halpern also rejects music skill regression based on aging; however, she did identify some music tasks, such as the ability to recognize a set of newly learned melodies, that do seem to indicate age-related decrements. The researcher concluded that there are many music cognitive tasks that even nonmusical older adults are well-equipped to succeed at and to enjoy.

Reminiscence is the recollection of past experiences or events. Research indicates that reminiscing can contribute to improved mental health among older adults (Cappeliez & O'Rourke, 2006). Cohen and Taylor (1998) examined functions of different types of reminiscence and found that types of reminiscence and amounts of reminiscence are related to clients' lifestyles and ages. Several researchers have examined the use of reminiscence music therapy sessions on recall and depressive symptoms and found that music can be beneficial in aiding reminiscence and has positive effects on mood (Ashida, 2000; Wylie, 1990). Reminiscing is a cognitive skill that remains fairly intact in older adults and is one that creates a sense of continuity by linking events of the past to the present. Karras (2001, 2005) and Karras and Hansen (2005) have developed materials particularly suitable for music therapists using reminiscence activities.

CONCLUSION

With healthcare at risk and unavailable to many citizens, wellness programs are becoming more popular and are adopting new approaches to meet the needs of contemporary society (Rotenberk, 2007). Research indicates that older adults are interested in wellness and that they are willing to make lifestyle changes in order to maintain their health (Campbell & Kreidler, 1994; Viverais-Dresler, Bakker, & Vance, 1995; White & Nezey, 1996). However, Campbell and Kreidler (1994) found that many older adults believe that good health is inherited and often out of their control. Such belief systems prevent many older adults from engaging in healthy practices such as exercise and wise nutritional choices. Older adults may need to be convinced of their own ability to influence their health in order to increase the benefits of wellness programs (Ghetti et al., 2008). By participating in wellness programs, older adults can exercise their personal responsibility to good health.

Music has the potential to enhance all areas of wellness programs. Music can serve as a motivator and a reward for engaging in many activities that promote general wellness. It also serves easily as a facilitator of socialization and physical activity—both important components of general wellness. Research has shown music therapy to be a valuable contributor to the health and wellness of older adults (Clair & Memmott, 2008; Roskam & Reuer, 1999). Music offers the older adult a familiar medium, and one that is invaluable in its flexibility and utility.

REFERENCES

American Music Therapy Association (AMTA). (2009). *AMTA member sourcebook*. Silver Spring, MD: Author.

Ashida, S. (2000). The effect of reminiscence music therapy session on changes in depressive symptoms in elderly persons with dementia. *Journal of Music Therapy, 37*, 170–182.

Banks, S., & Dinger, D. F. (2007). Behavioral and physiological consequences of sleep restriction. *Journal of Clinical Sleep Medicine, 3*(5), 519–528.

Batt-Rawden, K. B. (2006). Music: A strategy to promote health in rehabilitation? An evaluation of participation in a 'music and health promotion project.' *International Journal of Rehabilitation Research, 29*(2), 171–173.

Beckett, A. (1990). The effects of music on exercise as determined by physiological recovery heart rates and distance. *Journal of Music Therapy, 27*, 126–136.

Belgrave, M., & Darrow, A. A. (2007, November). *Effect of participation in intergenerational music activities on participants' cross-age attitudes, positive nonverbal behaviors and behaviors of engagement.* Presentation at the annual meeting of the American Music Therapy Association, Louisville, KY.

Bernardi, L., Porta, C., & Sleight, P. (2006). Cardiovascular, cerebrovascular and respiratory changes induced by different types of music in musicians and non-musicians: The importance of silence. *Heart, 92*(4), 445–452.

Bittman, B., Berk, L. S., Felten, D. L., Westengard, J., Simonton, O. C., & Pappas, J. (2001). Composite effects of group drumming music therapy on modulation of neuroendocrine-immune parameters in normal subjects. *Alternative Therapies in Health and Medicine, 7*(1), 38–47.

Bowers, J. (1998). Effects of intergenerational choir for community-based seniors and college students on age-related attitudes. *Journal of Music Therapy, 35*(1), 2–18.

Bradt, J., & Dileo, C. (2009). Music for stress and anxiety reduction in coronary heart disease patients. *Cochrane Database Systematic Reviews, 15*(2), CD006577.

Bruhn, K. T., & Clair, A. A. (1999, July). *Active music making and wellness.* Remo HealthRHYTHMS. Retrieved March 8, 2010, from http://www.remo.com/portal/pages/health_rhythms/library_article1.html

Buchhaupt, T. (2000). Music therapy as a treatment for chronic pain disorders: A case report. *Anasthesiologie, Intensivmedizin, Notfallmedizin, Schmerztherapie: AINS, 35*, 406–411.

Bugos, J. A. (2007). Individualized piano instruction enhances executive functioning and working memory in older adults. *Aging and Mental Health, 11*(4), 464–471.

Campbell, J., & Kreidler, M. (1994). Older adults' perceptions about wellness. *Journal of Holistic Nursing, 12*, 437–447.

Cappeliez, P., & O'Rourke, N. (2006). Empirical validation of a model of reminiscence and health in later life. *Journal of Gerontology: Psychological and Social Science, 61*, 237–244.

Cevasco, A. M., & Grant, R. E. (2003). Comparisons for different methods for eliciting exercise-to-music for clients with Alzheimer's disease. *Journal of Music Therapy, 40*, 41–56.

Christiansen, M. (2007). *Guitar for seniors.* Pacific, MO: Mel Bay.

Clair, A. A. (1996). *Therapeutic uses of music with older adults.* Baltimore: Health Professions Press.

Clair, A. A. (1998). *Active music making and wellness applications*. Unpublished manuscript, University of Kansas, Lawrence.

Clair, A. A. (2008). Music therapy and elderly populations. In W. Davis, K. Gfeller, & M. Thaut (Eds.), *Introduction to music therapy* (pp. 181–207). Silver Spring, MD: American Music Therapy Association.

Clair, A. A., & Memmott, J. (2008). *Therapeutic uses of music with older adults*. Silver Spring, MD: American Music Therapy Association.

Coffman, D. D. (2002). Music and quality of life in older adults. *Psychomusicology, 18*, 76–88.

Coffman, D. D., & Adamek, M. (1999). The contribution of wind band participation to quality of life of senior adults. *Music Therapy Perspectives, 17*, 27–31.

Coffman, D. D., & Adamek, M. (2001). Perceived social support of New Horizons Band participants. *Contributions to Music Education, 28*(1), 27–40.

Cohen, A., Bailey, B., & Nilsson, T. (2002). The importance of music to seniors. *Psychomusicology, 18*, 89–102.

Cohen, G., Perlstein, S., Chapline, J., Kelly, J., Firth, K. M., & Simmens, S. (2006). The impact of professionally conducted cultural programs on the physical health, mental health, and social functioning of older adults. *The Gerontologist, 46*, 726–734.

Cohen, G., & Taylor, S. (1998). Reminiscence and ageing. *Ageing and Society, 18*, 601–610.

Daly, J. (2005). *Evidence-based medicine and the search for a science of clinical care*. Berkeley, CA: University of California Press.

Darrow, A. A., Johnson, C. M., & Ollenberger, T. (1994). The effect of participation in an intergenerational choir on teens' and older persons' cross-age attitudes. *Journal of Music Therapy, 31*, 119–134.

Douglass, D. (1985). *Accent on rhythm: Music activities for the aged* (3rd ed.). St. Louis, MO: MMB Music.

Engen, R. L. (2005). The singer's breath: Implications for treatment of persons with emphysema. *Journal of Music Therapy, 42*, 20–48.

Foster, N. A., & Valentine, E. R. (2001). The effect of auditory stimulation on auto-biographical recall in dementia. *Experimental Aging Research, 27*, 215–228.

Frytak, J. R. (2000). Assessment of quality of life. In R. L. Kane and R. A. Kane (Eds.), *Assessing older persons: Measures, meaning, and practical applications* (pp. 200–236). New York: Oxford University Press.

Ghetti, C. M., Hama, M., & Woolrich, J. (2008). Wellness and music therapy. In A. A. Darrow (Ed.), *Introduction to approaches in music therapy* (2nd ed., 131–151). Silver Spring, MD: American Music Therapy Association.

Gibbons, A. C. (1982a). Musical Aptitude Profile scores in a non-institutionalized elderly population. *Journal of Research in Music Education, 30*, 23–29.

Gibbons, A. C. (1982b). A musical skill level self-evaluation in a non-institutionalized elderly population. *Activities, Adaptation & Aging, 3*(1), 61–67.

Gibbons, A. C. (1983). Primary measures of music audiation scores in an institutionalized elderly population. *Journal of Music Therapy, 20,* 21–29.

Gibbons, A. C. (1984). A program for non-institutionalized, mature adults: A description. *Activities, Adaptations, and Aging, 6,* 71–80.

Gibbons, A. C. (1988). A review of literature for music development/education and music therapy with elderly. *Music Therapy Perspectives, 5,* 33–40.

Grape, C., Sandgren, M., Hansson, L. O., Ericson, M., & Theorell, T. (2003). Does singing promote well-being? An empirical study of professional and amateur singers during a singing lesson. *Integrative Physiological and Behavioral Science, 38,* 65–74.

Gregory, D. (2002). Music listening for maintaining attention of older adults with cognitive impairments. *Journal of Music Therapy, 39,* 244–264.

Hagen, B., Armstrong-Esther, C., & Sandilands, M. (2003). On a happier note: Validation of musical exercise for older persons in long-term care settings. *International Journal of Nursing Studies, 40*(4), 347–357.

Halpern, A. R. (2002). Aging and memory for music: A review. *Psychomusicology, 18,* 10–27.

Hamburg, J., & Clair, A. A. (2003). The effects of a movement with music program on measures of balance and gait speed in healthy older adults. *Journal of Music Therapy, 40*(3), 212–226.

Hamburg, J., & Clair, A. A. (2004). The effects of a Laban-based movement program with music on measures of balance and gait in older adults. *Activities, Adaptation, & Aging, 28*(1), 17–33.

Hanser, S. S. (1990). A music therapy strategy for depressed older adults in the community. *Journal of Applied Gerontology, 9,* 283–298.

Hanser, S. B., & Thompson, L. W. (1994). Effects of a music therapy strategy on depressed older adults. *Journal of Gerontology, 49*(6), 265–269.

Harris, Y. (2007). Depression as a risk factor for nursing home admission among older individuals. *Journal of American Medical Directors Association, 8*(1), 14–20.

Hays, T. (2006). Facilitating well-being through music for older people with special needs. *Home Health Care Services Quarterly, 25*(3–4), 55–73.

Hays, T., Bright, R., & Minichiello, V. (2002). The contribution of music to positive aging: A review. *Journal of Aging and Identity, 7*(3), 165–175.

Hirokawa, E. (2004). Effects of music listening and relaxation instructions on arousal changes and the working memory task in older adults. *Journal of Music Therapy, 41,* 107–127.

Jensen, L. A., & Allen, M. N. (1994). A synthesis of qualitative research on wellness-illness. *Qualitative Health Research, 4*(4), 349–369.

Johnson, G., Otto, D., & Clair, A. A. (2001). The effect of instrumental and vocal music on the adherence to a physical rehabilitation exercise program with persons who are elderly. *Journal of Music Therapy, 38,* 82–96.

Johnson, J. E. (2003). The use of music to promote sleep in older women. *Journal of Community Health Nursing, 20*(1), 27–35.

Kamel, N. S., & Gammack, J. K. (2006). Insomnia in the elderly: Cause, approach, and treatment. *American Journal of Medicine, 119*(6), 463–469.

Karras, B. (2001). *Roses in December: Music sessions with older adults.* Mt. Airy, MD: ElderSong.

Karras, B. (2005). *Down memory lane: Topics and ideas for reminiscence groups* (2nd ed.). Mt. Airy, MD: ElderSong.

Karras, B., & Hansen, S. T. (2005). *Journey through the 20th century: Activities for reminiscing and discussion.* Mt. Airy, MD: ElderSong.

Koga, M., & Tims, F. (2001). The music making and wellness project. *American Music Teacher, 51*(2), 18–22.

Krout, R. E. (2006). Music listening to facilitate relaxation and promote wellness: Integrated aspects of our neurophysiological responses to music. *The Arts in Psychotherapy, 34*, 134–141.

Lai, H. L. (2004). Music preference and relaxation in Taiwanese elderly people. *Geriatric Nursing, 25*(5), 286–291.

Lai, H. L., & Good, M. (2005). Music improves sleep quality in older adults. *Journal of Advanced Nursing, 49*(3), 234–244.

Laukka, P. (2007). Uses of music and psychological well-being among the elderly. *Journal of Happiness Studies, 8*, 215–241.

Maratos, A. S., Gold, C., Wang, X., & Crawford, M. J. (2008). Music therapy for depression. *Cochrane Database Systematic Reviews, 23*(1), CD004517.

McBride, S., Graydon, J., Sidani, S., & Hall, L. (1999). The therapeutic use of music for dyspnea and anxiety in patients with COPD who live at home. *Journal of Holistic Nursing, 17*(3), 229–250.

McCaffrey, R., & Freeman, E. (2003). Effect of music on chronic osteoarthritis pain in older adults. *Journal of Advanced Nursing, 44*, 517–524.

McCaffrey, R., & Locsin, R. (2006). The effect of music on pain and acute confusion in older adults undergoing hip and knee surgery. *Holistic Nursing Practice, 20*(5), 218–224.

McKinney, C. H., Antoni, M. H., Kumar, M., Tims, F. C., & McCabe, P. M. (1997). Effects of guided imagery and music (GIM) therapy on mood and cortisol in healthy adults. *Health Psychology, 16*(4), 390–400.

Miller, M. P. (1991). Factors promoting wellness in the aged person: An ethnographic study. *Advances in Nursing Science, 13*(4), 38–51.

Mitchell, L. K., & McDonald, R. A. R. (2006). An experimental investigation of the effects of preferred and relaxing music listening on pain perception. *Journal of Music Therapy, 43*, 295–316.

Modesti, P. A., et al. (2008). *Daily sessions of music can reduce 24-hour ambulatory blood pressure in mild hypertension.* Presentation at the meeting of the American Society of Hypertension, Abstract 230.

Mornhinweg, G. C., & Voignier, R. R. (1995). Music for sleep disturbance in the elderly. *Journal of Holistic Nursing, 13*(3), 248–254.

O'Callaghan, C., & Grocke, D. (2009). Lyric analysis research in music therapy: Rationales, methods and representations. *The Arts in Psychotherapy, 36*(5), 320–328.

Okamoto, H., Stracke, H., Stoll, W., & Pantev, C. (2009). Listening to tailor-made notched music reduces tinnitus loudness and tinnitus-related auditory cortex activity. *Proceedings of the National Academy of Sciences, 107*(3), 1207–1210.

Olson, B. K. (1984). Player piano music as therapy for the elderly. *Journal of Music Therapy, 21*, 35–45.

Pelletier, C. L. (2004). The effect of music on decreasing arousal due to stress: A meta-analysis. *Journal of Music Therapy, 41*, 192–214.

Pierdomenico, S. D., Di Nicola, M., Esposito, A. L., Di Mascio, R., Ballone, E., Lapenna, D., & Cuccurullo, F. (2009). Prognostic value of different indices of blood pressure variability in hypertensive patients. *American Journal of Hypertension, 22*(8), 842–847.

Raglio, A., Bellelli, G., Traficante, D., Gianotti, M., Ubezio, M. C., Villani, D., & Trabucchi, M. (2008). Efficacy of music therapy in the treatment of behavioral and psychiatric symptoms of dementia. *Alzheimer Disease & Associated Disorders, 22*, 158–162.

Reuer, B. L., Crowe, B., & Bernstein, B. (2007). *Group rhythm and drumming with older adults: Music therapy techniques and multimedia training guide.* Silver Spring, MD: American Music Therapy Association.

Roskam, K., & Reuer, B. (1999). A music therapy wellness model for illness prevention. In C. Dileo (Ed.), *Music therapy and medicine: Theoretical and clinical applications* (pp. 139–147). Silver Spring, MD: American Music Therapy Association.

Rotenberk, L. (2007). Wellness programs gain popularity, take on new approaches. *Hospitals & Health Networks, 81*(8), 30.

Sadovsky, R. (1998). Prevalence and recognition of depression in elderly patients. *American Academy of Family Physicians, 57*(5), 1096–1097.

Shapiro, D. W., Lasker, R. D., Bindman, A. B., & Lee, P. R. (1993). Containing costs while improving quality of care: The role of profiling and practice guideline. *Annual Review of Public Health, 14*, 219–241.

Siedliecki, S. L., & Good, M. (2006). Effect of music on power, pain, depression and disability. *Journal of Advanced Nursing, 54*, 553–562.

Sloboda, J. A., & O'Neill, S. A. (2001). Emotions in everyday listening to music. In P. N. Juslin & J. A. Sloboda (Eds.), *Music and emotion: Theory and research* (pp. 415–430). Oxford, England: Oxford University Press.

Smith, D. S., & Lipe, A. W. (1991). Music therapy practices in gerontology. *Journal of Music Therapy, 28*, 193–210.

Stull, J. E. (2005). *The effects of familiar music, unfamiliar music, and no music on face-name recall in aging adults.* Unpublished master's thesis, Florida State University, Tallahassee.

Suzuki, M., Kanamori, M., Nagasawa, S., Tokiko, I., & Takayoki, S. (2007). Music therapy-induced changes in behavioral evaluations, and saliva chromogranin a and immunoglobulin a concentrations in elderly patients with senile dementia. *Geriatrics and Gerontology International, 7*(1), 61 –71.

Teel, C. S., Carson, P., Hamburg, J., & Clair, A. A. (1999). Developing a movement program with music for older adults. *Journal of Aging and Physical Activity, 7*, 400–413.

Twiss, E., Seaver, J., & McCaffrey, R. (2006). The effect of music listening on older adults undergoing cardiovascular surgery. *Nursing Critical Care, 11*(5), 224–231.

U.S. Public Health Service. (2009). *Report of the Surgeon General's conference on older adults and mental health: A national section agenda.* Washington, DC: U. S. Department of Health and Human Services. Retrieved December 15, 2009, from http://www.surgeongeneral.gov/library/mentalhealth/home.html

VanderArk, S., Newman, I., & Bell, S. (1983). The effects of music participation on quality of life of the elderly. *Music Therapy, 3*, 71–81.

VanWeelden, K., & Whipple, J. (2004). Effect of field experiences on music therapy students' perceptions of choral music for geriatric wellness programs. *Journal of Music Therapy, 41*, 340–352.

Verghese, J., Lipton, R., Katz, M., Hall, C., Derby, C., Kuslansky, G., & Buschke, H. (2003). Leisure activities and the risk of dementia in the elderly. *The New England Journal of Medicine, 248*, 2508–2516.

Viverais-Dresler, G. A., Bakker, D. A., & Vance, R. J. (1995). Elderly clients' perceptions: Individual health counseling and group sessions. *Canadian Journal of Public Health, 86*, 234–237.

Watt, D., Verma, S., & Flynn, L. (1998). Wellness programs: A review of the evidence. *Canadian Medical Association Journal, 158*, 224–230.

Weideman, D. A. (1986). *The effect of reminiscence and music on movement participation level of elderly care-home residents.* Unpublished master's thesis, The University of Kansas, Lawrence.

White, J., & Nezey, I. O. (1996). Project wellness: A collaborative health promotion program for older adults. *Nursing Connection, 9*, 21–27.

Wininger, S. R., & Pargman, D. (2003). Assessment of factors associated with exercise enjoyment. *Journal of Music Therapy, 40*(1), 57–73.

Wise, G. W., Hartmann, D. J., & Fisher, B. J. (1992). Exploration of the relationship between choral singing and successful aging. *Psychological Reports, 70*, 1175–1183.

Wylie, M. E. (1990). A comparison of the effects of old familiar songs, antique objects, historical summaries, and general questions on the reminiscence of nursing-home residents. *Journal of Music Therapy, 27*, 2–12.

Zelazny, C. M. (2001). Therapeutic instrumental music playing in hand rehabilitation for older adults with osteoarthritis: Four case studies. *Journal of Music Therapy, 38*, 97–113.

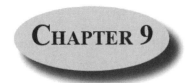

CHAPTER 9

CLINICAL APPLICATIONS FOR WELLNESS

Singing relieves stress and helps my voice to stay strong. I love coming to choir and singing with my new friends. —Mrs. C.

I always wanted to learn to play guitar, but never had the time. Now I do and I love it. My grandkids are proud of me too. Whenever they come over, they always want to hear me play. —Mr. S.

This chapter contains clinical applications that promote wellness in older adults. These applications are organized for staff with no music training, staff or volunteers with some musical training or music skills, and board-certified music therapists with advanced skills in music and working with older adults. The chapter is divided into the four focus areas of general wellness programs: lifelong learning and wellness, physical wellness, cognitive wellness, and emotional wellness. The clinical applications in each focus area are hierarchical and begin with activities that can be carried out by general staff, then staff or volunteers who are also musicians, and, finally, music therapists. The learning activities contain target behavior, advanced preparation required, implementation directions, and helpful websites or possible materials. At the conclusion of the chapter is a bibliography on older adults' musical preferences and appropriate song repertoire for older adults.

Important Note: A useful website to use throughout the applications is one that lists the top songs by year and decade: http://www.musicimprint.com/Chart.aspx?id=C000097. Many of the activities suggest selecting songs from seniors' teen or young adult years, generally the 20s, and downloading the songs from iTunes. Determining the appropriate year or decade of songs that represent seniors' teen or young adult years requires calculating the seniors' mean age (collective age divided by the number of seniors).

FOCUS AREA 1: ADDRESSING LIFELONG LEARNING WITH MUSIC

Clinical Application 3.1 ——————————————————————————————

Target Behavior: Discussing music and its relevance to life experiences

Music: Music listening

Level 1—General Staff

Activity Name: "What Music Means to Me"

Advanced Preparation: Survey participants as to who has an interest in music, particularly listening to music. Be sure to reassure them that expressing an interest in music does not necessarily mean training in music or an interest in performing music. After determining participants' mean age, select 10 songs from their teen or young adult years and download from iTunes.

Activity Direction: Gather participants and provide them with a playlist of the selected songs. Guide discussion by asking the following questions:

1. For how many of these songs can you sing the first line?
2. What were you doing in life when one or more of these songs was popular?
3. Do any of these songs have a special meaning for you?

Provide lyrics for any songs in which the participants express an interest. Play the recordings of those songs and allow participants to quietly follow the lyrics or sing along. After each song, ask the participants to think about the lyrics. Guide discussion by asking the following questions:

1. What meaning do you find in the lyrics?
2. Has the meaning of the lyrics changed for you over the years?
3. Do you think your interpretation of the lyrics is influenced by life events? If so, which ones?

Target Behavior: Discussing music and its relevance to life experiences

Music: Music listening

Level 2—Volunteer Musician

Activity Name: "What Music Means to Me"

Advanced Preparation: Survey participants as to who has an interest in music, particularly listening to music. Be sure to reassure them that expressing an interest in music does not necessarily mean training in music or an interest in performing music. After determining participants' mean age, select 10 songs from their teen or young adult years and download music from Sheet Music Plus: http://www.sheetmusicplus.com/.

Activity Direction: Gather participants and provide them with a playlist of the selected songs. Guide discussion by asking the following questions:

1. For how many of these songs can you sing the first line?
   (Accompany participants as they sing.)
2. What were you doing in life when one or more of these songs was popular?
3. Do any of these songs have a special meaning for you?

Provide lyrics for any songs in which the participants express an interest. Perform those songs on the piano or guitar and allow participants to quietly follow the lyrics or sing along. After each song, ask the participants to think about the lyrics. Guide discussion by asking the following questions:

1. What meaning do you find in the lyrics?
2. Has the meaning of the lyrics changed for you over the years?
3. Do you think your interpretation of the lyrics is influenced by life events? If so, which ones?

As you play the accompaniments, lead the participants in singing the songs that were discussed to close the session.

Target Behavior: Discussing music and its relevance to life experiences

Music: Music listening

Level 3—Board-Certified Music Therapist

Activity Name: "Lyric Analysis"

Advanced Preparation: Survey participants as to who has an interest in music, particularly listening to music. Be certain to reassure them that expressing an interest in music does not necessarily mean an interest in performing music. After determining participants' mean age, select 10 songs from their teen or young adult years and download music from Sheet Music Plus: http://www.sheetmusicplus.com/. Transpose songs so they are in appropriate keys for senior singers.

Activity Direction: Gather participants and provide them with a playlist of the selected songs. Guide discussion by asking the following questions:

1. Were you able to sing the first line to any of these songs?
   (Accompany participants as they sing.)
2. What were you doing in life when one or more of these songs was popular?
3. Do any of these songs have a special meaning for you?

Provide lyrics for any songs in which the participants express an interest. Perform those songs on the piano or guitar and allow participants to quietly follow the lyrics or sing along. After each song, ask the participants to think about the lyrics. Guide discussion by asking the following questions:

1. What meaning do you find in the lyrics?
2. Has the meaning of the lyrics changed for you over the years?
3. Do you think your interpretation of the lyrics is influenced by life events? If so, which ones?
4. What emotion do you think the composer was trying to convey?
5. Identify for participants the musical elements that help to convey a certain emotion (tempo, key, texture, harmonic structure, dynamics, etc.).

Based upon the discussion, adapt lyrics, music, or musical style to convey new meanings and/or style preferences of participants. For participants who may not be interested in singing, provide them with instruments that are appropriate to the style of the music. Demonstrate an appropriate ostinati for them to play while others sing. Use rhythmic speech to match the ostinati so participants have a verbal cue to remember the ostinati.

Clinical Application 3.2

Target Behavior: Discussing music and musical performances

Music: Music listening

Level 1—General Staff

Activity Name: "It's Show Time!"

Advanced Preparation: Call local churches or community choir groups. Invite them to perform at your facility. If there is a university with a music program, invite students who are preparing recitals to do a final dress rehearsal at your facility. High school choirs often do musicals. Invite the choir members to practice solos or chorus numbers from the musical for your residents.

Activity Direction: Plan a program for the local residents. Be sure to advertise within the facility, prepare a written program of talent show participants, and invite friends and family. After the performance, invite residents to discuss the performances. Possible questions are:

1. What was your favorite musical performance? Why?
2. What time period were the musical selections from?
3. What emotions did you feel when you listened to the music? What emotions do you think the performers were trying to convey? Were they successful?
4. Did the music remind you of any events in your life?

Target Behavior: Performing and discussing music

Music: Music listening and performing

Level 2—Volunteer Musician

Activity Name: "It's Show Time!"

Advanced Preparation: Survey participants or residents to determine those who enjoy singing or who have played an instrument. Bring together all the individuals who expressed an interest in music.

1. Write the names of all individuals who enjoy singing. Compile a list of their favorite songs. Ask them to rank order the list of songs according to their preference. Take the top 5 to 8 songs and find the lyrics online at http://www.songlyrics.com/. Prepare songs sheets for the participants. Go to iTunes and find karaoke recordings of the

songs. Song downloads are generally 99 cents each. If a pianist is available, go to http://www.sheetmusicplus.com/ and download the music for the selected songs. Transpose keys if necessary. Determine if there are any individuals who would like to sing a solo. Miming humorous songs can also be fun for individuals who do not sing.

2. Write the names of all individuals who have played an instrument and determine if they still have the instrument. For those who do, ask them to prepare one piece for a talent show. Play chords or the written accompaniments with the instrumentalists. If possible, play duets with the instrumentalists.

Activity Direction: Plan a talent show of the local residents. Be sure to advertise within the facility, schedule regular rehearsals, prepare a written program of talent show participants, and invite friends and family.

Target Behavior: Performing and discussing music

Music: Music listening and performing

Level 3—Board-Certified Music Therapist

Activity Name: "It's Show Time!"

Advanced Preparation: Survey participants or residents to determine those who enjoy singing or who have played an instrument. Bring together all the individuals who expressed an interest in music.

1. Write the names of all individuals who enjoy singing. Compile a list of their favorite songs. Ask them to rank order the list of songs according to their preference. Take the top 5 to 8 songs and find the lyrics online at http://www.songlyrics.com/. Prepare songs sheets for the participants. Go to http://www.sheetmusicplus.com/ and download the music for the selected songs. Transpose keys if necessary or order in a specific key. Write alternate parts for individuals who are capable of singing harmony. Teach these parts to those who wish to sing harmony. Determine if there are any individuals who would like to sing a solo. Miming humorous songs can also be fun for individuals who do not sing. Write an arrangement for appropriate rhythm instruments.

2. Write the names of all individuals who have played an instrument and determine if they still have the instrument. For those who do, ask them to prepare one piece for a talent show. Play chords or the written accompaniments with the instrumentalists. If possible, play duets with the instrumentalists.

3. Write an arrangement that includes the instruments that others in the group play, or an arrangement for appropriate rhythm instruments as an accompaniment to the soloists.

4. Provide lessons to participants who may need remedial work on their instruments or who want to advance their musical skills.

Activity Direction: Plan a talent show of the local residents. Be sure to advertise within the facility, schedule regular rehearsals, prepare a written program of talent show participants, and invite friends and family.

Clinical Application 3.3

Target Behavior: Writing and discussing song lyrics

Music: Writing song lyrics to familiar melodies

Level 1—General Staff

Activity Name: "Songs by YOU!"

Advanced Preparation: Survey participants as to their interest in music, particularly listening to and singing songs. Be certain to reassure them that expressing an interest in music does not necessarily mean they must be a musician. After determining participants' mean age, select 10 songs from their teen or young adult years and download from iTunes. Lyrics can be found at http://www.songlyrics.com/. Prepare copies of the lyrics. Be sure to enlarge if necessary. Listen to the songs and invite older adults to sing along.

Activity Direction: Prepare lyrics sheets of the songs with selected words omitted and replaced with a blank space or line. Be sure to select words from different word classes (verbs, nouns, pronouns, proper names, etc.). Ask the participants to replace the omitted words with words of their own from the same word classes. Download a karaoke version of the song from iTunes and have participants sing their newly "composed song."

Target Behavior: Writing and discussing song lyrics

Music: Writing song lyrics to familiar melodies

Level 2—Volunteer Musician

Activity Name: "Songs by YOU!"

Advanced Preparation: Survey older adults as to their interest in music, particularly listening to and singing songs. Be certain to reassure them that expressing an interest in music does not necessarily mean they must be a trained musician. After determining participants' mean age, select 10 songs from their teen or young adult years and download from iTunes. Lyrics can be found at http://www.songlyrics.com/. Prepare copies of the lyrics. Be sure to enlarge if necessary. Listen to the songs and invite older adults to sing along.

Activity Direction: Ask participants to identify the emotion of the song and the message of the song. Using their own words, ask participants to paraphrase the song lyrics, or write their own lyrics for each line, matching the emotions and meaning of the song. For example, with Eddy Arnold's song, "Mother" (*"M" is for the million things she gave me, "O" means only that she's growing old, "T" is for the tears she shed to save me, "H" is for her heart of purest gold, "E" is for her eyes with love-light shining, "R" means right and right she'll always be.*

Put them all together; they spell MOTHER, a word that means the world to me), ask participants to identify different words to go with each letter of the word *mother*, or to write a song called "Father" using the same melody. Download a karaoke version of the song from iTunes or play the song, and have participants sing their newly "composed song."

Target Behavior: Writing and discussing song lyrics

Music: Writing song lyrics to familiar melodies

Level 3—Board-Certified Music Therapist

Activity Name: "Songs by YOU!"

Advanced Preparation: Survey older adults as to their interest in music or poetry, particularly listening to and singing songs or writing poetry. Be sure to reassure them that expressing an interest in music or poetry does not necessarily mean they must be a musician or a poet.

Activity Direction: Tell participants they are going to write a song—collectively. Carry out the following steps on a large paper tablet, overhead, or white board.

Step 1: Pick a topic, particularly one relevant to their lives. It can be about a season, friends, health, family, a mood, etc.

Step 2: Write all the words the group can think of related to the selected topic.

Step 3: Using the words in step 2, write sentences related to the topic. Arrange sentences in a logical order. Try to include rhyming words when possible.

Step 4: Decide on a tempo appropriate to the topic. Is it thoughtful, cheerful, silly, etc.?

Step 5: Take each line and ask participants if they have a melody for that line in their heads. If not, propose one to the group.

Step 6: Continue until the all the lines have a melody assigned and record each line on a digital recorder.

If the therapist can do it during the initial session, play chords to accompany participants while they sing. If not, prepare an accompaniment for the next session and record the song. Depending on the therapist's skills, he or she can write harmony parts and an instrumental accompaniment for participants to play or for a MIDI keyboard. Have participants share their song with others at the facility. Record and make CD copies to send to family members.

Clinical Application 3.4

Target Behavior: Listening to rhythms and replicating rhythms

Music: Playing rhythm instruments

Level 1—General Staff

Activity Name: "Finding the Groove"

Advanced Preparation: Survey participants as to songs they remember and like. If they have difficulty remembering the names of songs, determine participants' mean age, select 3 to 5 songs from their teen or young adult years, and download from iTunes. Purchase ½-inch dowel rods from the local hardware store and have them cut into 12-inch lengths, or order rhythm sticks from West Music: http://www.westmusic.com/.

Activity Direction:

1. Using the rhythm sticks, ask half of the group to play the steady beat of a song selected by the group. Ask the other half of the group to play the melodic rhythm of the song (the rhythm that follows the words/lyrics).
2. Play the song again and switch the playing assignment for each group.
3. As the leader, play the rhythm of one line of the lyrics. Ask participants what line in the song matches the rhythm you played. Go around the room and ask each person to play the rhythm of one line while the others guess the line.
4. As an art activity, participants can paint and decorate the sticks.

Target Behavior: Listening to rhythms and replicating rhythms

Music: Playing rhythm instruments

Level 2—Volunteer Musician

Activity Name: "Finding the Groove"

Advanced Preparation: Download songs or music with an obvious beat from iTunes. Military marches or swing music are good genres for rhythm activities. Purchase ½-inch dowel rods from the local hardware store and have them cut into 12-inch lengths.

Activity Direction: Pair participants and place in two lines facing each other, either in chairs facing each other or across a narrow table facing each other. Ask participants to find the steady beat in the music. With a partner, model a simple 4-beat pattern using your own and your partner's sticks. For example, tap your own sticks against each other two times, and then your right stick against your partner's right stick two times. Have participants create their own 4-beat pattern with their partner. Ask each pair of participants to demonstrate their rhythm. Starting at the one end, have each pair play their rhythm—going from one pair to the next without stopping. Do again with the recorded music or music you play on the piano or guitar. Playing the piano or guitar allows you, the leader, to modify the tempo. Be sure to select music that is not too fast. Once the pairs' rhythm routines are secure, pick up the tempo. As a follow-up activity, create rhythms based on 8-beat patterns.

Target Behavior: Listening to rhythms and replicating rhythms

Music: Playing rhythm instruments

Level 3—Board-Certified Music Therapist

Activity Name: "Finding the Groove"

Advanced Preparation: Select music from military marches or other music with a strong, steady beat. Use commercial rhythm sticks or purchase ½-inch dowel rods from the local hardware store and have them cut into 12-inch lengths. Incorporate other rhythm instruments or hard plastic stadium cups.

Activity Direction: Write a specific rhythm accompaniment to the selected tune. Begin with quarter notes and quarter rests only. Make or use commercial rhythm cards. To chant the rhythms, use *ta* for quarter notes and *ti ti* for two eighth notes, the word *rest* for rests, or any familiar word set (such as fruits) to illustrate rhythmic syllabication. Musicians often use *ta* and *ti* for quarter and eighth notes, but there is no magic in the syllables. Learners just need some syllable chant that matches the note durations. Gradually incorporate two barred eighth notes, half notes, and sixteenth notes. Examples of fruit names to illustrate rhythmic syllabication include: quarter note = *pear*, two eighth notes = *ap-ple*, four sixteenth notes = *wa-ter-mel-on*, quarter rest = *rest*, half note = *gra-pe*. Icons of the fruit or the fruit names can be placed beneath the notes as a cue for chanting the rhythm. Have the participants play the rhythm cards to the music using traditional rhythm instruments. Participants can also use hard plastic stadium cups to create their own rhythms. Participants can create rhythms by tapping the cups, tapping them on a table, passing them from one hand to the other, and passing them to the person seated next to them. This is a rhythm activity that can be executed with participants seated around a table. Rather than creating the rhythm accompaniment, the music therapist can use commercial rhythm arrangements, but still use them to accompany music that is selected by the group of older adults. One example of rhythm arrangements is *Essential Rhythm Activities for the Music Classroom*: http://www.amazon.com/Essential-Rhythm-Activities-Music-Classroom/dp/0739050931.

FOCUS AREA 2: ADDRESSING PHYSICAL WELLNESS WITH MUSIC

Clinical Application 3.5

Target Behavior: Exercising upper body and manipulating objects

Music: Listening to music and moving scarves or streamers

Level 1—General Staff

Activity Name: "Movin' and Groovin'"

Advanced Preparation: Survey participants as to songs they remember and like. After determining participants' mean age, select 3 to 5 songs from their teen or young adult years and download from iTunes. Make or purchase chiffon scarves or streamers on a stick.

Activity Direction: Ask participants to move scarves or streamers to the rhythm or melody of the music. Shorter streamers are easier for older adults to move. Those with no physical limitations can move longer streamers and they are often more attractive. There are commercial CDs for streamer musical activities. One can be found at http://www.westmusic.com/ProductDetails.aspx?prodid=850285

Target Behavior: Exercising the upper body

Music: Listening and moving to music

Level 2—Volunteer Musician

Activity Name: "Movin' and Groovin'"

Advanced Preparation: Watch a video of competitive wheelchair dancers for movement ideas—http://www.youtube.com/watch?v=cJ9NqyChCA0—or show to the group to promote chair dancing. Commercial DVDs can be found for chair dancing as well. A popular one is *Jodi Stolove's Chair Dancing* available at Amazon.com.

Activity Direction: Using the materials listed above, select movements appropriate to the physical abilities of your group. Set the movements to the preferred music of the older adults. Encourage partner movements for socialization purposes and to promote positive touch behaviors. Positive touch behaviors are limited among many older adults—often resulting in "skin hunger."

Target Behavior: Exercising the upper body

Music: Listening and moving to music

Level 3—Board-Certified Music Therapist

Activity Name: "Movin' and Groovin'"

Advanced Preparation: Purchase *Motivating Moves* by Janet Hamburg from:

Parkinson Foundation of the Heartland
8900 State Line Road, Suite 320
Overland Park, KS 66206
Cost: $19.95 for a VHS videotape, DVD, PAL or SECAM videotape, plus shipping.
Priority shipping is available.

Activity Direction: *Motivating Moves* was originally designed for individuals with Parkinson's disease but is equally appropriate for all older adults. *Motivating Moves* is an approach to exercise that emphasizes coordination, balance, flexibility, postural alignment, diaphragmatic breathing, spatial awareness, and dynamic movement range.

Motivating Moves teaches you how to improve your strength and reduce your risk of injury. Exercises in *Motivating Moves* require coordinating movements of the upper and lower body and right and left sides. The movements are varied in tempo, spatial direction, dynamic qualities, complexity of phrasing, and according to which body parts are most active.

Clinical Application 3.6

Target Behavior: Exercising upper body and sequential memory

Music: Music listening and hand jive

Level 1—General Staff

Activity Name: "Born to Hand Jive"

Advanced Preparation: Purchase the soundtrack or download from iTunes, *Hand Jive* from the movie *Grease*. Watch the video *Hand Jive*: http://www.youtube.com/watch?v=yj4UVp9aKl4. This video will give you the instructions for the hand jive movements.

Activity Direction: Teach the group the hand jive movements above. Add on each new hand jive movement after the previous movement is secure. Practice first without the music, gradually getting faster and faster. After the group feels comfortable with the movements, use the music and encourage the group to move their upper body to the music as they execute the hand movements. Depending on participants' ages, some are likely to remember this song from the 1950s.

Target Behavior: Exercising the upper body and sequential memory

Music: Music listening, singing, and hand jive

Level 2—Volunteer Musician

Activity Name: "Mexican Hand Clapping Song"

Advanced Preparation: Purchase or download for 99 cents the "Mexican Hand Clapping Song" from Ella Jenkin's *This Is Rhythm*: http://www.amazon.com/Mexican-Hand-Clapping-Song/dp/B000S4BD2W. Learn the song and hand clapping.

Activity Direction: Teach the "Mexican Hand Clapping Song." Accompany the group on the piano or guitar. By accompanying the group rather than using the recording, you can adjust the tempo of the song to their abilities. After the group is secure, use the recording to accompany the group.

Target Behavior: Exercising the upper body and sequential memory

Music: Music listening, singing, and hand jive

Level 3—Board-Certified Music Therapist

Activity Name: "Clappin' and Jivin'"

Advanced Preparation: Watch the video *Patty Cake*: http://www.youtube.com/watch?v=TwdaLphAhdA. Break down the steps in the video or create your own "Patty Cake" sequence. You may also want to watch a slower *Patty Cake*: http://www.youtube.com/watch?v=HrV8bhdNlvE&feature=related.

Activity Direction: Pair participants. Teach a clapping sequence to the group. Ask them to create their own chants, or use the one above: "Bake me a cake as fast as you can." They can also create their own Patty Cake sequence. You can ask the group to change their tempos throughout the sequence as the first video above, or you can accompany the group on the piano to help keep the tempo even and from getting progressively faster.

Clinical Application 3.7

Target Behavior: Exercising upper body

Music: Singing and moving

Level 1—General Staff

Activity Name: "YMCA"

Advanced Preparation: Download "YMCA" by the Village People. You can see the original 1978 version of "YMCA" at http://www.youtube.com/watch?v=CS9OO0S5w2k.

Activity Direction: Listen to the song above. This is a popular wedding dance where the full arms are used to create the letters Y-M-C-A when the letters are sung. During all other parts of the song, have the group clap their hands. Ask the group if they can think of any other letters they can create with their full arms.

Target Behavior: Exercising upper body

Music: Singing and moving

Level 2—Volunteer Musician

Activity Name: "A Boy and a Girl"

Advanced Preparation: Go to the following website: http://kristinhall.org/songbook/Motions.html. It is a collection of songs with motions. There are many you can use, but check for age appropriateness. A good one to start with is "A Boy and a Girl." The chords are provided with suggestions for the motions. If you don't know the melody, you can create one to fit the chords provided.

Activity Direction: Go over the lyrics using the suggested motions, or have the group create their own motions. Encourage big movements that will exercise participants' upper body.

Target Behavior: Exercising upper body

Music: Creating and playing instruments

Level 3—Board-Certified Music Therapist

Activity Name: "One Dark and Stormy Night"

Advanced Preparation: You will need a large white board or paper chart and several sets of rhythm instruments.

Activity Direction: As a group, create a short story that starts with "One dark and stormy night . . ." Write the story on the white board as the group creates it. As the leader, you can write the first line. For example, "One dark and stormy night, a black cat crossed in front of a young boy walking down the street." Ask participants to add the next line, and so forth. After the story is created, ask participants to select instruments that match the story line. For example, for "One dark and stormy night," ask one participant to play a thunder tube and another to play a rain stick or to slap his or her thighs to simulate rain. A slap stick can be used for lightning. For the boy walking down the street, ask someone to play temple blocks or a wood block in a walking tempo. For the cat, ask someone to make vocal sounds. Continue the story, selecting instruments to accompany selected lines of the story.

Clinical Application 3.8

Target Behavior: Exercising lower body

Music: Listening, singing, and moving

Level 1—General Staff

Activity Name: "Can Can"

Advanced Preparation: Download the music to "Can-Can" from the musical *Can-Can.*

Activity Direction: Explain to the group the history of the Can-Can. *Can-Can* is a musical with music and lyrics by Cole Porter and a book by Abe Burrows. The story concerns the showgirls of the Montmartre dance halls during the 1890s. You can find out more information on the Internet. Afterwards, play the music and have the group make up steps using only their legs in a seated position. Be sure to include a good number of leg kicks and side-to-side steps.

Target Behavior: Exercising the entire body

Music: Listening, singing, and moving

Level 2—Volunteer Musician

Activity Name: "Hey, Big Spender"

Advanced Preparation: Download the song "Hey Big Spender," either the sheet music or from iTunes. Have the following video prepared: http://www.youtube.com/watch?v =WAJ58w4r5kk. Each participant should have a chair without arms.

Activity Direction: Listen to the song and watch the video for movement ideas. Divide your participants into three groups. Have each group create three movements using their chairs. Have each group showcase their moves. Vote and select one group for the day who will teach their moves to the rest of the participants. This process can continue until you have enough moves for the entire song.

Target Behavior: Exercising the entire body

Music: Listening, singing, and moving

Level 3—Board-Certified Music Therapist

Activity Name: "Cupid Shuffle"

Advanced Preparation: Download the song "Cupid Shuffle."

Activity Direction: Listen to the song and watch the video: http://www.youtube.com/ watch?v=iJQKBk4oDr4. This is an easy and repetitive dance. Even though it is a hip-hop dance, many older adults have learned this dance and enjoyed doing it. A music therapist can break down the steps and accompany on the guitar to match the tempo capabilities of the dancers.

FOCUS AREA 3: ADDRESSING COGNITIVE WELLNESS WITH MUSIC

Clinical Application 3.9 ─────────────────────────

Target Behavior: Exercising sequential memory

Music: Playing percussion instruments

Level 1—General Staff

Activity Name: "What's the Rhythm of Your Name?"

Advanced Preparation: Purchase a small group of rhythm instruments. Some instruments can be made inexpensively, such as egg shakers, sand blocks, or rhythm sticks.

Activity Direction: Lead participants in a music game designed to enhance memory. Participants will sit in a circle and a variety of small percussion instruments will be in the center of the circle. The first participant will choose an instrument from the center and play it in rhythm while chanting his or her name. The rhythm can be the syllables of his or her name, for example, *O-liv-i-a* or *Tom-mie.* The next participant will copy what the last person did, then add his or her own instrument and name afterward. The game progresses around the circle and participants must remember the previous instruments and names in order and then add their own. Teamwork will be encouraged if a participant has trouble remembering the sequence. If the group is too large to remember all the names and rhythms, the group and instruments can be divided into smaller groups.

Target Behavior: Exercising short-term functional memory

Music: Singing songs

Level 2—Volunteer Musician

Activity Name: "Going to the Store"

Advanced Preparation: Large paper chart, overhead, or white board. Piano or guitar music for selected songs preferred by group participants.

Activity Direction: The group writes a hypothetical grocery list of 10 selected items on the chart or white board. Help the group set the list to a familiar tune. The group practices the list of items set to the familiar tune. Participants then write down as many grocery items as they can remember. Discuss with the group the use of music and chants as a mnemonic device.

Target Behavior: Exercising short-term functional memory

Music: Singing songs

Level 3—Board-Certified Music Therapist

Activity Name: "Musical Names"

Advanced Preparation: Download the list of song titles with people's names: http://www.philbrodieband.com/music_song_titles_names.htm. Possible song examples for women are "Goodnight Irene," "Once in Love with Amy," "K-K-K-Katy," "Annie's Song," "Barbara Ann," "Eleanor Rigby," "Georgia on My Mind," and "Peggy Sue." Possible song examples for men include "Danny Boy," "Tom Dooley," "Ben," "Brian's Song," "Johnny Be Good," "Frankie and Johnny," "Hit the Road, Jack," and "Big Bad John." Take photos from magazines of 5 women and 5 men. Make a set of photos for each member of the group.

Activity Direction: Pass out the list of songs and a set of photos to each participant. Decide on one song to represent each photo. Practice singing the songs while participants study the photos. Afterwards pair up partners to work in teams and remember the names and songs of each photo as you hold them up.

Clinical Application 3.10

Target Behavior: Exercising long-term memory

Music: Remembering and reading the lyrics to familiar songs

Level 1—General Staff

Activity Name: "Missing Words"

Advanced Preparation: Purchase *Sing-A-Long Golden Oldies*: http://www.ideamusic.org/ books_oldies.htm. Prepare song sheets of selected songs with certain words omitted and blanks inserted for the missing words.

Activity Direction: Divide the group into teams and ask them to fill in as many blanks as they can. The group with the most blanks filled in wins the game.

Target Behavior: Exercising long-term memory

Music: Listening to and singing familiar songs

Level 2—Volunteer Musician

Activity Name: "Missing Words"

Advanced Preparation: Purchase *Sing-A-Long Golden Oldies*: http://www.ideamusic.org/ books_oldies.htm. Prepare song sheets of selected songs with certain words omitted and blanks inserted for the missing words.

Activity Direction: Divide the group into teams and ask them to fill in as many blanks as they can. The group with the most blanks filled in wins the game. Sing the songs after the group has filled in the missing words. Find recordings of the selected songs on iTunes and ask participants to name the artist of the songs.

Target Behavior: Exercising long-term memory

Music: Listening to and singing familiar songs

Level 3—Board-Certified Music Therapist

Activity Name: "Missing Words"

Advanced Preparation: Purchase *Sing-A-Long Golden Oldies*: http://www.ideamusic.org/ books_oldies.htm. Prepare song sheets of selected songs with certain words omitted and blanks inserted for the missing words.

Activity Direction: Divide participants into teams. Sing and play songs selected from *Sing-A-Long Golden Oldies*. Periodically stop and ask participants in one team to sing the next word. Go back and forth between the two teams. Therapists can also stop and ask participants to sing the next phrase, or ask participants to quietly sing the song in their heads (audiating) and sing only the first or last word of every phrase. Therapists will likely need to point to the group at the time they are to sing and remind them to stop afterwards and sing only "in their heads."

Clinical Application 3.11

Target Behavior: Exercising short-term, sequential, functional memory

Music: Singing and moving, creating music

Level 1—General Staff

Activity Name: "Singing and Moving to Your Name"

Advanced Preparation: Have participants sit in a circle.

Activity Direction: Ask participants to sing their first names and to create simple hand movements to match what they are singing. If participants have difficulty matching movements to their sung names, suggest simple hand jive movements. Go around the circle and ask participants to repeat previous sung names and hand movements, and then to add their own.

Target Behavior: Exercising short-term, functional memory

Music: Singing and listening

Level 2—Volunteer Musician

Activity Name: "Singing and Moving to Your Name"

Advanced Preparation: Ask participants to sit in a circle.

Activity Direction: Sing or chant a short phrase about each participant. Phrases can include the color of the participant's hair, facial expression, clothing, etc. For example, "Susie is sitting there with a smile on her face. Isn't she sweet?" or "Bill is wearing brown pants. Can he dance?" Sing the phrases again immediately, leaving out key words and asking participants to fill in the blanks.

Target Behavior: Exercising short-term, functional memory

Music: Singing and listening

Level 3—Board-Certified Music Therapist

Activity Name: "The Name Game" and "The Clapping Song"

Advanced Preparation: Learn to play and sing Shirley Ellis's "The Name Game," and Shirley Ellis's "The Clapping Song."

Activity Direction:
1. Watch the video of Shirley Ellis singing "The Name Game": http://www.youtube.com/watch?v=5MJLi5_dyn0. Sing and teach the song to the group, incorporating their names one by one.

2. Watch the video of Shirley Ellis singing "The Clapping Song": http://www.youtube.com/watch?v=bgnCB7oni8o&NR=1. Sing and teach the song to the group, breaking down the clapping exercises and slowly increasing the tempo.

Clinical Application 3.12

Target Behavior: Reminiscence and recalling memories

Music: Listening and responding to music

Level 1—General Staff

Activity Name: "Name That Tune"

Advanced Preparation: Select songs from the CD *The Melody Lingers On* by Bill Messenger (2004), ISBN 1-892132-47-8, Venture Publishing, Inc.

Activity Direction: Divide participants into teams. Play selected songs from the CD *The Melody Lingers On*. Teams get points for every song they can name and an extra point if they can remember the artist who made it famous. Participants share any memories associated with the songs, or the times they were popular.

Target Behavior: Reminiscence and recalling memories

Music: Listening and responding to music

Level 2—Volunteer Musician

Activity Name: "Oh, Yes, That Reminds Me . . ."

Advanced Preparation: Select songs from the CD *The Melody Lingers On* by Bill Messenger (2004), ISBN 1-892132-47-8, Venture Publishing, Inc.

Activity Direction: Each song in the sing-along section of the CD and text (Part 2) is preceded by background information on the song, which may be used by the group leader as a means to prompt and facilitate conversation and reminiscing. Direct the group in singing each song after listening to the background information and participating in reminiscence.

Target Behavior: Reminiscence and recalling memories

Music: Listening and responding to music

Level 3—Board-Certified Music Therapist

Activity Name: "Telling My Story"

Advanced Preparation: Select songs from the CD, *The Melody Lingers On* by Bill Messenger (2004), ISBN 1-892132-47-8, Venture Publishing, Inc.

Activity Direction: The book contains original piano and guitar arrangements of 20 of the best-loved songs from the turn of the century. Play songs and write arrangements for participants to accompany on rhythm instruments. After singing and playing selected songs, participants can engage in associated movement and reminiscence activities. After a reminiscence period, create a CD of each participant's "story" with appropriate improvised background music. CDs can be gifts to participants' families.

FOCUS AREA 4: ADDRESSING EMOTIONAL WELLNESS WITH MUSIC

Clinical Application 3.13

Target Behavior: Discussion of music's meaning in the lives of older adults

Music: Music listening

Level 1—General Staff

Activity Name: "Music and the Young@Heart"

Advanced Preparation: Find NBC's *The Today Show* segment on the documentary "Young@Heart," a choir of (much) older adults who spend their free time singing rock tunes for very appreciative audiences across the country and around the world. The segment can be found at http://content.foxsearchlight.com/inside/node/2599, or the full video can be purchased online at http://www.amazon.com/Young-Heart-Joe-Benoit/dp/B001BBAVKQ.

Activity Direction: The segment illustrates the important role music performance can play in the lives and emotional health of older adults. Have participants view the segment and then lead participants in a discussion of music's meaning in their lives and in the lives of the characters portrayed in the *Today Show* segment. Possible questions to prompt discussion are:

1. What did music do for the members of Young@Heart?
2. Has music ever provided similar meaning in your lives?
3. How did the Young@Heart members deal with the death of their fellow choir member?
4. Do you think music making provided comfort to them when they were dealing with the loss of friends?
5. How might you use music in similar ways?
6. Were their musical performances perfect? Did it seem to matter to the audience?
7. Why do you think the audience enjoyed their music so?

Target Behavior: Discussion of music's meaning in the lives of young teens

Music: Music listening

Level 2—Volunteer Musician

Activity Name: "Forever Young"

Advanced Preparation: Invite teen musicians from a local high school choir or school service organization to come and perform or play recordings of their favorite songs. Ask them to present songs representing both slow and fast tempos and a variety of styles (pop, country, hip hop, etc.).

Activity Direction: Have high school students perform or play recordings of their favorite songs (approximately 20–30 minutes of music). Ask the students to talk about the artists and what the lyrics mean to them. After the students leave or while they are still there, ask the older adults to talk about the music they heard. Possible questions are:

1. Did you like any music selections?
2. Why did you prefer these selections?
3. Were you surprised by any of the music selections?
4. What did you think of the students' musical discussion?
5. Were there any musical attributes that were common to the music of your own teen years?

Provide song sheets of selected music the teens presented and ask older adults to listen or sing as you play the music. Lyrics can be found at http://www.songlyrics.com/ and sheet music can most likely be found at http://www.sheetmusicplus.com/.

Target Behavior: Performing for others, community integration

Music: Singing and performing

Level 3—Board-Certified Music Therapist

Activity Name: "Rock of Ages"

Advanced Preparation: Contact a local high school, community college, or university choir director and invite them to participate in an intergenerational rock choir. Send them the video website of Young@Heart: http://content.foxsearchlight.com/inside/node/2599 and that of the Intergenerational Rock Choir at Florida State University: http://www.theallegro.com/news/2008_04_23.html.

Activity Direction: Organize members into a rock choir that rehearses each week. Arrange music as needed using local church, community, or university musicians for the band, or use karaoke recordings. Possible program numbers are:

- "In My Life" by the Beatles (with slides of older adults in their younger years, wedding pictures, family pictures, etc.)
- "Forever Young" by Rod Stewart or "Forever Young" by Neil Young as a closing number
- "Imagine" by the Beatles (with slides from rehearsals)
- "We Will Rock You" by Queen as a possible opening number
- "Old Time Rock & Roll" by Bob Seger as a possible opening number
- "My Generation" by The Who

- "Stayin' Alive" by the Bee Gees
- "I Feel Good" by James Brown
- "Stand by Me" by John Lennon
- "Lean on Me" by Bill Withers
- Possible dance numbers: "Twist and Shout," "Hound Dog," "Jailhouse Rock," "Blue Suede Shoes"
- Possible audience sing-a-longs: "Proud Mary," "Let It Be," "Joy to the World," "I Wanna Hold Your Hand"

Clinical Application 3.14

Target Behavior: Discussing the relationship between mood and music

Music: Music listening

Level 1—General Staff

Activity Name: "Mood Music"

Advanced Preparation: Select a variety of music from commercially available CDs, particularly examples of (1) easy listening music, sometimes called elevator music or music for relaxation; and (2) dance music. For dance music, select music that represents participants' preferred music: swing, country, jazz, or pop.

Activity Direction: Listen to excerpts of the selected music, starting with the music for relaxation and moving to the dance music. On a large writing chart, or white board, ask participants to write words that they think of as they listen to the music. Try to guide participants to select adjectives that might indicate how the music makes them feel. If they offer words that remind them of events in their life, you may also want to make the activity a reminiscence activity as well as a discussion about music and feelings. Lead a discussion about how the music makes participants feel and how they might purposefully use the music in their daily lives to relax, to go to sleep, and to meditate, or to exercise, to dance, to lift their spirits, etc.

Target Behavior: Changing mood from negative to positive

Music: Music listening and playing

Level 2—Volunteer Musician

Activity Name: "Drumming Up"

Advanced Preparation: Organize participants in a circle with various drums. Incorporate other percussion instruments if you do not have enough drums.

Activity Direction: Briefly discuss the role of musical tempo as an indication of mood. Ask participants if there is music they listen to when they are happy or when they are sad. Ask them to identify the tempos of the music, either fast or slow. Go around the circle and ask participants to improvise on the drums to indicate their mood. Lead the group in a drumming circle that matches each ostinati to participants' individual improvisation (mood). After everyone is drumming, add the final ostinati that is upbeat and engaging. To determine if moods have changed, quickly go around the circle and ask participants again to improvise on the drums to indicate their mood.

Target Behavior: Changing mood from negative to positive

Music: Music listening and singing

Level 3—Board-Certified Music Therapist

Activity Name: "Iso-Principle"

Advanced Preparation: Based on the age of the individual or group participants, select songs from their young adult years. Select four songs ranging from the slowest tempo to the fastest tempo. A good resource for this activity can be found at http://www.severing.nu/music/. This is a list of the greatest hits from the 40s to the present.

Activity Direction: Utilizing the Iso-Principle, organize the four songs moving from the tempo that seems to match the mood of participants to the mood that you are trying to create. For the purposes of wellness programs, the principle generally serves to bring seniors up, starting with a slow tempo song and gradually moving through the songs to the fastest tempo song. Encouraging participants to sing and to clap, as the songs pick up in tempo, assists in achieving mood change.

Clinical Application 3.15

Target Behavior: Music-assisted relaxation

Music: Music listening

Level 1—General Staff

Activity Name: "Time to Go to Bed"

Advanced Preparation: Purchase one of the following CDs available at most Borders stores:

1. Pachelbel's *Canon with Ocean Surf*
2. *A Day without Rain* by Enya
3. Vivaldi's *Four Seasons* by Music for Relaxation

The following CDs by Steven Halpern are available at most Barnes and Noble stores:
1. *Sleep Soundly*
2. *Effortless Relaxation*
3. *Letting Go of Stress*

Activity Direction: Offer a relaxation session in the early evening. Use the CDs above to guide the participants in deep breathing and relaxation exercises. Use the following as an example of a verbal guide:

Preparation: *Get into a relaxed position. . . . Close your eyes. Take a very deep breath. Begin to relax and let the concerns of the day fall away. Focus on the rhythm of your own breathing as a sense of peace fills you. The sense of calm centers you. It feels so good to take this time to unwind. The peacefulness begins to fill your body. Each part of your body unwinds—beginning in your feet. Your toes, arches, and heels begin to relax. The sense of peace moves upward and begins to loosen the muscles of your legs, your knees, then thighs and hips. Go limp. Your lower body is totally relaxed—feet, knees, thighs, hips, muscles in your fingers and hands. Relax as you concentrate on your breathing. Slow breaths in and out. Your forearms loosen up, then your upper arms. The peaceful sense moves to the base of your spine and moves up your back into your shoulders—they relax easily. The muscles in your neck and scalp smooth out, as the tension slips away. Your back and arms are totally relaxed. The calmness slides into the muscles of your face and jaw. Your mouth falls open a bit as you again become aware of your breathing, low and deep. The last remaining tension in your body flows out with your breath. Take a few slow breaths quietly to clear your mind.*

(http://www.allaboutcounseling.com/imagery_relaxation_technique.htm)

Target Behavior: Reminiscence

Music: Music accompaniment

Level 2—Volunteer Musician

Activity Name: "My Life"

Advanced Preparation: Ask participants to write a short story about some meaningful event in their life.

Activity Direction: Read through the stories and select music to accompany the stories. For example, if a story is about a wedding, use the Wedding March or other traditional wedding music as the background music, or for a story about a special Christmas, use traditional Christmas music as the background music. For a war story, use popular songs, such as "When Johnny Comes Marching Home Again." For stories about children, use children's songs, etc.

Prepare a program of story sharing. As participants read their story into a microphone, play the appropriate music in the background. Background music adds to the emotional impact of the stories. If the volunteer or staff musician is an accomplished pianist, he or she may be able to improvise appropriate background music.

Target Behavior: Reminiscence

Music: Music accompaniment

Level 3—Board-Certified Music Therapist

Activity Name: "My Travels"

Advanced Preparation: Ask participants to write a short story about travels to other countries or to special venues in the United States.

Activity Direction: Read through the stories and select music to accompany the stories. For example, if a story is about a trip to the Grand Canyon, use the *Grand Canyon Suite* by Frede Grofé; a trip to New York, use "New York New York" or "New York State of Mind"; a trip to the Rocky Mountains, use "Rocky Mountain High" or *Night on Bald Mountain*; a trip to Paris, use "I Love Paris," or "Under Paris Skies." A helpful list of songs with numerous different countries in the titles can be found at http://www.songfacts.com/category:songs _with_names_of_countries_in_the_title.php.

Prepare a program of story sharing. As participants read their story into a microphone, play the appropriate music in the background. Background music adds to the emotional impact of the stories. If you are a pianist or guitarist, you may be able to improvise appropriate background music.

Clinical Application 3.16

Target Behavior: Reminiscence, sharing stories of friendship

Music: Music listening

Level 1—General Staff

Activity Name: "Acts of Friendship"

Advanced Preparation: Select songs from the following list and download from iTunes:

- "You've Got a Friend" by James Taylor
- "Thank You for Being a Friend" by Andrew Gold
- "Lean on Me" by Bill Withers
- "I'll Be There for You" by The Rembrandts
- "That's What Friends Are For" by Dionne Warwick
- "Wind Beneath My Wings" by Bette Midler
- "With a Little Help from My Friends" by The Beatles
- "Stand by Me" by Ben E. King
- "He Ain't Heavy, He's My Brother" by The Hollies
- "You Got a Friend in Me" by Randy Newman
- "I'll Stand by You" by The Pretenders
- "You're My Best Friend" by Queen
- "Bridge Over Troubled Water" by Simon and Garfunkle

Activity Direction: Play several of the songs listed above. Allow participants to follow along with song sheets. Lyrics can be found at http://www.lyrics.com. Use songs to stimulate discussion about friendship. Ask each participant to share an incident with a friend, or an act of kindness by a stranger. Ask participants to share acts of friendship extended to them and acts of friendship they extended to others.

Target Behavior: Discussion, altering mood

Music: Music listening

Level 2—Volunteer Musician

Activity Name: "Let's Get Up!"

Advanced Preparation: Select songs that have "happiness" or "smiling" as the theme of the song. Examples are:

Happy:
- "Don't Worry, Be Happy"
- "Come On, Get Happy"
- "Happy Days Are Here Again"
- "So Happy Together"
- "You Made Me So Very Happy"
- "Oh, Happy Day"
- "Put on a Happy Face"

Smile:
- "When You're Smiling"
- "Smile a Little Smile for Me"
- "Smile"
- "When Irish Eyes Are Smiling"
- "I Love Your Smile"
- "Your Smiling Face"
- "You're Never Fully Dressed without a Smile"

Activity Direction: Play several of the songs listed above. Allow participants to follow along with song sheets. Lyrics can be found at http://www.lyrics.com. Use songs to stimulate discussion about reasons to be happy or to smile. Ask participants to share something that makes them happy or makes them smile. Conclude with reasons participants have to be happy (friendship, good weather, family, faith, etc.).

Target Behavior: Discussion, songwriting, altering mood

Music: Songwriting

Level 3—Board-Certified Music Therapist

Activity Name: "Personal Songs of Joy"

Advanced Preparation: Have a large writing chart, white board, or pad of paper.

Activity Direction: Starting with just a few older adults, ask each person his or her reasons for being happy or for smiling. Write down the reasons under each person's name. Allow participants to elaborate and take notes. Using your notes, compose a personal song of joy for each individual. Melodies can be original or lyrics can be "piggybacked" onto the melody of one of the individual's favorite songs. Write out lyric sheets and chord sheets for each song. Share the songs with individuals and ask them to sing along. Record the songs and make a

CD for each individual. Title the CDs after the person, such as *George's Personal Song of Joy*.

Everyone, old or young, needs to be reminded of the many reasons to be happy, especially when life gets difficult. As you give the CDs to the individuals, suggest that they listen and sing along when they go through difficult times. Encourage them to share their personal songs of joy with others.

ANNOTATED BIBLIOGRAPHY

Appropriate Song Repertoire for Geriatric Populations

Gibbons, A. C. (1977). Pop music preferences of elderly persons. *Journal of Music Therapy, 14*, 180–189.

A basic premise in music therapy practice is that most adults prefer music of their young adult years to music of other life periods, and that preferred music is more likely to promote participation in music therapy activities than non-preferred music. It is also quite commonly assumed that elderly adults tend to prefer sedative to stimulative musical experiences. In order to test these assumptions about elderly persons' musical preferences, a study was conducted ($N = 60$) to determine (a) whether elderly people tend to prefer music that was popular in their young adult years to music that was popular later in their lives, and (b) whether elderly people prefer stimulative to sedative music. Results of the study indicated that elderly persons strongly prefer popular music of their young adult years to popular music of life periods after young adulthood ($p < .001$). Results also indicated that there were no statistically significant differences in preferences for sedative or stimulative music. However, the raw data showed that elderly persons tend to prefer stimulative to sedative music in all age categories. The study supports the music therapy premise that adults prefer music of their young adult years, but refutes the notion that elderly persons tend to prefer sedative to stimulative music. If music preference is a factor in successful music experiences for elderly adults, then popular music of young adult years may more likely promote successful experience than popular music of later life periods.

Jonas, J. L. (1991). Preferences of elderly music listeners residing in nursing homes for art music, traditional jazz, popular music of today, and country music. *Journal of Music Therapy, 28*, 149–160.

The purpose of this study was to investigate seniors' comparative music preference for four generic styles including art music, country music, popular music of today, and traditional jazz. The study also attempted to identify certain variables that have an effect on preference. Sixty-three subjects with a mean age of 82.5 from four nursing homes in the South Central Michigan area participated in the study. An interview and musical preference test were administered to the subjects individually. The listening test consisted of 16 music selections, four from each style. The seniors judged how much they liked the selections on a scale from 1 to 5, with 5 indicating greatest preference. Results indicated that country music style was preferred the most, followed by traditional jazz, art music, and, lastly, popular music. Variables that were found to affect preference were education level, community size in which the seniors grew up, and music training outside the school setting.

Lathom, W., Peterson, M., & Havlicek, L. (1982). Musical preferences of older people attending nutrition sites. *Educational Gerontology, 8*, 155–165.

A hundred and four subjects, aged 55 years or older, listened to musical excerpts and stated their preferences among the eight musical styles represented. Subjects generally preferred patriotic, big band, and religious music, and were least fond of symphonic, operatic, and folk music. Preferences were closely related to educational level and previous musical experience. Implications for music therapy and recreational activities with older clients were discussed.

Moore, R., Staum, M., & Brotons, M. (1992). Music preferences of the elderly: Repertoire, vocal ranges, tempos, and accompaniments for singing. *Journal of Music Therapy, 29*, 236–252.

Three studies investigated musical preferences of elderly persons for song repertoire, vocal range, tempo, and background accompaniment of live and recorded songs. Data were collected from 514 persons over 65 years old with various physical, mental, and emotional disabilities, as well as higher functioning individuals in independent living settings. Results indicated that (a) patriotic and popular songs and hymns are preferred over folksongs; (b) vocal ranges average 19 semitones, or F3 to C5, for women and nearly an octave lower for men; (c) slower and moderate tempos are preferred to faster tempos; and (d) live and recorded chordal accompaniments are preferred to recorded melodic line or synthesized accompaniments. Guidelines for clinical applications include the following: (a) use music that geriatric populations enjoy since they clearly discriminate preferences, (b) possess a broad repertoire of songs, and (c) be able to accompany songs on a chordal instrument using suitable ranges for older voices and moderate tempos. Research on the use of music with geriatric individuals is limited. Exhaustive searches of the published material on this topic are available and indicate that, although interest in the area of gerontology is increasing, much research is still necessary (Galloway, 1975; Prickett, 1988). Music programs have been surveyed in several nursing homes.

Prickett, C. A., & Bridges, M. S. (2000). Song repertoire across the generations: A comparison of music therapy majors' and senior citizens' recognitions. *Journal of Music Therapy, 37*, 196–204.

This study examined whether a basic song repertoire of folk-type melodies that can be accompanied with principal triads exists in the senior citizen population and compared this repertoire with that of music therapy students. An audiotape of the tunes of 25 standard songs, assumed in previous research to be known by everyone who has finished sixth grade, was played for undergraduate music therapy students ($N = 78$) and for healthy, active senior citizens ($N = 78$). None of the senior citizens had received any music therapy services, although many were involved in music activities such as the senior choir at church. Music therapy majors identified significantly more tunes than did the older listeners. Further analysis indicated that there is a good deal of overlap in the repertoires of these two groups. Sixteen tunes were recognized by 80% of the therapy students; 10 songs were recognized by 80% of the seniors; the 10 songs identified by the seniors were 10 of the top 11 identified by the college students ("Kumbaya" was not known by the older listeners). Six songs could not be named by 50% of the students; 7 songs could not be named by 50% of the seniors; these two lists contained 5 common selections ("Oh, Shenandoah," "Kookaburra," "Down in the Valley," "Shalom Chaverim," and "Tinga Layo"). Given the growth of the senior segment of the American population, the expansion of services for them, and the popularity of including music activities among these services, it would appear that music therapy students' basic knowledge of a repertoire of songs that are known to older people and that can easily be accompanied with principal triads is adequate, even though the range of songs that could be identified was broad (11–24) and the mean correctly named was merely 70.82% of a set that other investigators, teachers, and professional organizations have said represent a minimal repertoire for all citizens beyond the sixth grade.

VanWeelden, K., & Cevasco, A. M. (2007). Repertoire recommendations by music therapists for geriatric clients during singing activities. *Music Therapy Perspectives, 25*, 4–12.

Little is known about the actual repertoire music therapists use with geriatric clients during singing activities, particularly whether the repertoire choices represent the young adult years of persons categorized as seniors, as previous researchers have suggested. Therefore, the purposes of this study were (a) to determine specific repertoire music therapists are using with geriatric clients during singing activities in the music styles of popular, patriotic, hymn, folk, and musicals; and (b) to determine what decades their repertoire choices represented. Surveys were sent to 455 music therapists who worked with geriatric persons. Of these, 151 music therapists returned the survey, creating a 33% return rate. A combined total of songs (*N* = 1,688) were recommended within the five music styles. Results found popular music was the style category with the greatest number of song recommendations, followed by folk songs, songs from musicals, hymns, and patriotic songs, respectively. A complete list of the repertoire is included.

UNIT IV
MUSIC THERAPY
IN
INTERGENERATIONAL
PROGRAMMING (IG)

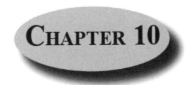

CHAPTER 10

Introduction to Intergenerational Programming and Music Therapy

The students were very generous because they volunteered after school when they could have been doing something more fun like games. Time after school is precious. —Mrs. E.

My grand friend and I have the same birthday. Tomorrow I'm turning 10 and she will turn 99. Wow. —Jasmine

This chapter contains an overview of intergenerational programming. Included in the overview is a history of why intergenerational programs were created, the typical models of intergenerational programs, and the benefits afforded to younger and older persons who participate in intergenerational programs. The reader will also be introduced to the use of music as an effective intervention in intergenerational programs. The information provided in this introduction will serve as the framework for the next two chapters pertaining to intergenerational programming, which includes a review of the literature and evidence-based music interventions for general staff, volunteer musicians, and music therapists to employ in various intergenerational settings.

Decreased Intergenerational Interactions

Today we live in an age-segregated society. There is limited contact between younger and older generations due to spatial and cultural segregation. Spatial segregation has occurred because living situations for older adults have changed. At one time in our history, it was common for older adults to live with their adult children and young grandchildren in a multigenerational household; however, such close living arrangements no longer exist for many families. Only 4% of older adults live in the same home with their adult children. Adult children do not always reside in the same city or state as their elderly parents, and, consequently, an increasing number of older adults are moving into adult living communities (Administration on Aging, 2007; Newman & Smith, 1997). With an increase in the number of senior living facilities and senior center programs, older adults' social networks and interactions usually occur with their peers. Younger generations' academic and social interactions occur with their peers throughout the school day and during after-school extracurricular activities (Haber & Short-Degraff, 1990; Hagestad & Uhlenberg, 2006; Powell & Arquitt, 1978; VanderVen, 1999).

Decreased intergenerational interactions contribute to cultural segregation between younger and older generations. Differences in dress, preferred music, leisure activities, and lexicons all contribute to how each generation experiences the world and their ability to relate to other generations that are different from themselves. The age, spatial, and cultural segregation experienced by younger and older generations has often resulted in misconceptions and stereotypes. Younger generations may believe that all older adults are ill and live in nursing homes, and older persons may believe that younger generations are undependable and lazy (Hagestad & Uhlenberg, 2006; Powell & Arquitt, 1978).

INTERGENERATIONAL PROGRAMS

Intergenerational programming is an effective way to bridge the generation gap by engaging younger and older generations in structured activities. Intergenerational programs provide an opportunity for individuals from both generations to relate to each other. The majority of research in intergenerational settings has been conducted with children and older adults. Engaging these two generations in meaningful interactions is fitting due to the social and emotional benefits afforded to both generations. Children benefit by becoming the recipients of older adults' nurturing, attention, and love, which is a necessary part of child development. Older adults gain purpose, meaning, and the opportunity to be connected to society by serving in a nurturing role. As intergenerational program research has grown, the younger generation has been expanded to include adolescents and college-age young adults (Aday, Rice, & Evans, 1991; Hagestad & Uhlenberg, 2006; Kaplin & Larkin, 2004; Karasik & Wallingford, 2007; Peacock & O'Quin, 2006; Powell & Arquitt, 1978; VanderVen, 1999).

Younger generations that are often involved in intergenerational programs are typically developing preschoolers, elementary-age children, adolescents, and college-age young adults, as well as young persons who are at-risk and have learning and developmental disabilities. Older adults who participate in intergenerational programs consist of individuals 65 years or older with varying physical and cognitive functioning levels. Intergenerational programs engage both generations in structured activities to decrease negative cross-age attitudes. Activities employed in intergenerational programs have included choirs, mentoring programs, weekly visits, and pen-pal and reading programs (Cote, Mosher-Ashley, & Kiernan, 2002; Darrow, Johnson, & Ollenberger, 1994; Dellmann-Jenkins, Fowler, Lambert, Fruit, & Richardson, 1994; Dunkle & Mikelthun, 1983; Kaplin & Larkin, 2004; Meshel & McGlynn, 2004).

It is believed that intergenerational programs are successful because individuals in both generations have needs that can be met through interactions inherent in multi-age activities. Intergenerational programs meet these needs because the foundation of any type of interpersonal interaction is social, though sometimes the task of an intergenerational group is academic as well as social—such as improving math skills through mentoring programs, or fostering prosocial behaviors like sharing and cooperating with others. Other objectives of intergenerational programs have included improving the self-esteem of elementary-age children, increasing adolescents' knowledge of the aging cycle, encouraging young adults to work in gerontological-related careers, fostering positive cross-age interactions, and enhancing older adults' psychosocial well-being (Cote et al., 2002; Cummings, Williams, & Ellis, 2002; Dellmann-Jenkins,

Lambert, & Fruit, 1991; Hill, 2007; Lowenthal & Egan, 1991; Kassab & Vance, 1999; Marx, Hubbard, Cohen-Mansfield, Dakheel-Ali, & Thein, 2005; Underwood & Dorfman, 2006). For young people to be successful in life, they must develop a variety of social skills as they age. For older people to age and maintain their emotional well-being, they must not be isolated or forgotten.

Needs of children, adolescents, and young adults are different and thus drive the objectives of and activities employed in intergenerational programs. The activities employed in intergenerational programs become more sophisticated as the age of the younger person increases. For example, music is a common activity used in many intergenerational programs. However, the function of the music changes because the skills required of adolescents and young adults to complete music activities are more advanced than the skills needed by young children. The body of research conducted in intergenerational settings is growing; however, the majority of this research focuses on the benefits afforded to the younger generation (Cote et al., 2002; Dellmann-Jenkins et al., 1994; Femia, Zarit, Blair, Jarrott, & Bruno, 2008; Kassab & Vance, 1999), with only a few studies focusing on the benefits older adults receive from these interactions (Newman, Karip, & Faux, 1995; Underwood & Dorfman, 2006; Ward, Kamp, & Newman, 1996).

MODELS OF INTERGENERATIONAL PROGRAMS

There are four models of intergenerational programs: (1) younger and older generations engaged in recreational activities; (2) younger and older generations engaged in combined learning programs; (3) older generations serving younger generations; and (4) younger generations serving older generations. Younger persons of all ages and older adults of varying ability levels have participated in leisure activities together through arts and crafts projects, music, and games. Younger and older generations learning new information or skills together are often a part of intergenerational classrooms, where younger and older generations are students together. In a community service program, the older adults serving younger generations model provides opportunities for older adults to share a skill or talent that they possess. The younger generations serving older generations model allows the older adults to learn something new such as computers or other forms of technology from younger generations (Gamliel, Reichental, & Eyal, 2007).

The model used to create an intergenerational program depends on the age, needs, and ability levels of both generations. These variables contribute to the diversity found among intergenerational programs. Intergenerational programs involving preschool-age children and older adults are created with a younger and older generation recreational model and an older adult serving younger person model. An intergenerational daycare program is one way to combine preschool-age children and older adults in recreational activities. Intergenerational daycare facilities are shared site programs in which services are provided for both generations throughout the day. Children attending these programs are typically between the ages of 6 weeks and 4 years of age. Older adults attending these programs are individuals who have cognitive and physical abilities that require them to attend an adult daycare program. Throughout the day there are opportunities for structured and unstructured interactions between children and older adults. The older adults serving preschoolers model is usually employed to improve the academic and social skills of the children. Older adults can promote reading readiness and assist with development and maintenance of prosocial behaviors, such as sharing and cooperation. Intergenerational programs involving elementary-age children, high school adolescents, and college-age young adults with older persons have used all four models to structure interactions. Examples of intergenerational programs involving children, adolescents, and young adults interacting with older adults include gardening projects; performing arts groups such as dance, theatre, or visual arts; academic tutoring; and younger generations leading older adults in choir rehearsals or walking programs to maintain and improve physical and psychosocial well-being (Ames & Youatt, 1994; Hamilton et al., 1999; Jarrott, Gigliotti, & Smock, 2006; Lowenthal & Egan, 1991; Peacock & O'Quin, 2006; Stremmel, Travis, Kelly-Harrison, & Hensley, 1994; VanWeelden & Whipple, 2004; Vernon, 1999; Whitehouse & Whitehouse, 2005).

Both younger and older generations receive many benefits from participating in intergenerational programs. Both generations experience purposeful interactions and, as a result, discover how to relate to one another. The interactions between the generations can also result in cross-age friendships and companionship. As a result of participation in intergenerational programs, younger generations have improved their school attendance, aging attitudes, and attitudes toward community service (Abrams & Giles, 1999; Karasik & Wallingford, 2007; Peacock & O'Quin, 2006; Stremmel et al., 1994; VanderVen, 1999; Zeldin, Larson, Camino, & O'Connor, 2005). Older adults have benefited from participation in intergenerational programs by having an increased sense of well-being, decreased isolation, and increased feelings of usefulness (Abrams & Giles, 1999; Kaplin & Larkin, 2004; Lindquist, 1986; Saltz, 1989; VanderVen, 1999).

CROSS-AGE ATTITUDES AND INTERACTIONS

An individual's attitude toward another is formed by three components: feelings toward, knowledge of, and interactions with another person (Williams & Nussbaum, 2001). In our society today, misconceptions and negative attitudes between younger and older generations often exist because of decreased interactions. Children may believe that all older adults are sick, frail, and live in nursing homes. Older adults may think that children and adolescents today are more disrespectful or lazy than they were when they themselves were young. The primary objective of most intergenerational programs is to decrease negative cross-age attitudes through increased positive interactions. The majority of research with younger generations has focused on promoting positive attitudes toward aging and older persons, whereas only a limited number of studies have examined older adults' attitudes toward younger generations. Results of such studies have provided mixed findings. Some studies have shown that cross-age attitudes improved after participation in an intergenerational program, whereas some studies have shown that attitudes became more negative or did not change (Corbin, Kagan, & Metal-Corbin, 1987; Corbin, Metal-Corbin, & Barg, 1989; Cummings et al., 2002; Femia et al., 2008; Lynott & Merola, 2007; Middlecamp & Gross, 2002; White, 2001). Although some researchers found that children and adolescents held negative views toward aging after participating in intergenerational programs, the younger generations reported that they enjoyed interacting with the older adults in the intergenerational programs (Barton, 1999; Corbin et al., 1987; White, 2001).

Intergenerational programs have also been created to improve younger persons' interactions with older adults. Interacting with older adults provides an opportunity for young children to improve social behaviors such as sharing, helping, caring and cooperating with others. Additionally, young persons have become more socially adept as a result of becoming more comfortable and willing to interact with older persons. Adding children to adult programs often increases older persons' participation and engagement in activities. Older adults are often more engaged in program activities with children than when they participate in activities with only older adults (Giglio, 2006; Leitner, 1981; Newman & Ward, 1992/1993; Ward et al., 1996). Research reveals that older adults in various stages of decline have received benefits from their interactions with young people in intergenerational programs (Ward et al., 1996).

OLDER ADULTS' PSYCHOSOCIAL WELL-BEING

Many intergenerational programs are beneficial to older adults because the structure of the programs provides them with opportunities to engage in meaningful activities. In programs with children, older adults often serve as teachers or mentors and are able to engage in meaningful activities that can contribute to their self-esteem and quality of life; however, this role changes with interactions that include young adults. Intergenerational programs for older and young adult participants involve both groups interacting in adult-related activities such as exercise programs, reminiscing through oral history, or choirs. The interactions in these settings provide opportunities for the formation of adult friendships and interactions (Bowers, 1998; Dellmann-Jenkins et al., 1994; Herrmann, Sipsas-Herrmann, Stafford, & Herrmann, 2005; Newman, Morris, & Streetman, 1999; Saxon & Etten, 2002; Underwood & Dorfman, 2006). In studies where researchers have measured psychosocial well-being, older adults have shared that intergenerational programs provide improvements in their overall quality of life, productivity, and life satisfaction. Participation in intergenerational programs provides an opportunity for older adults to give back to others, feel useful, and decrease their social isolation (Proller, 1989; White, 2001).

Older adults who have declines that require higher levels of care often move to assisted living facilities or nursing homes, or attend adult daycare centers (Administration on Aging, 2007). The psychosocial needs of individuals living in care facilities are similar to older adults in the community. However, the age-related declines that occur in older persons living in aging facilities can affect the number of meaningful activities in which they can participate, thus often leaving them socially isolated. Participation in intergenerational programs provides older adults with opportunities for social interactions and purposeful activities.

MUSIC-BASED INTERGENERATIONAL PROGRAMS

Music is an activity used frequently in intergenerational programs. Music, of some style or genre, is enjoyed by all age groups and is familiar to all people. People experience music everyday, whether it is waking to music, singing along to a favorite song on the radio, or hearing a catchy jingle in a television commercial. Music is also used to structure other daily activities, such as exercising or completing chores. Music can also be used to trigger memories of events or individuals. The song "Happy Birthday" may cause a person to remember a special birthday, or the song "Can I Have This Dance?" may bring memories of couples' first dance at their wedding. The flexibility of music—its simplicity or complexity—allows both younger and older generations to participate in music-based intergenerational programs.

Empirical research in music-based intergenerational programs has been conducted with older adults who live in residential programs and the community, with younger participants including infants, elementary-age children, high school adolescents, and college-age young adults (Belgrave & Darrow, 2010; Bowers, 1998; Darrow et al., 1994; St. John, 2008). Music-based programs have combined community-dwelling older adults with high school adolescents and college-age young adults in intergenerational choirs that use the music of both generations. Older adults in community and retirement living facilities often participate in intergenerational music programs that include interventions such as instrument playing, singing, and moving to music, and academic and social skills training. Studies utilizing music-based intergenerational groups have shown a change in cross-age attitudes, an increase in children's willingness to interact with older adults, an increase in spontaneous nonverbal behaviors of older adults, and an improvement in orientation and level of alertness for older adults when interacting with children (Belgrave & Darrow, 2010; Bowers, 1998; Darrow et al., 1994; Giglio, 2006; Newman & Ward, 1992/1993; St. John, 2008). The following chapter will provide a more in-depth account of the literature pertaining to the benefits younger and older generations receive when they participate in intergenerational programs.

REFERENCES

Abrams, J., & Giles, H. (1999). Intergenerational contact as intergroup communication. *Child & Youth Services, 20*(1/2), 203–217.

Aday, R. H., Rice, C., & Evans, E. (1991). Intergenerational partners project: A model linking elementary students with senior center volunteers. *The Gerontologist, 31*, 263–266.

Administration on Aging. (2007). *A profile of older Americans: 2007.* Washington, DC: Author.

Ames, B. D., & Youatt, J. P. (1994). Intergenerational education and service programming: A model for selection and evaluation of activities. *Educational Gerontology, 20*, 755–764.

Barton, H. (1999). Effects of an intergenerational program on the attitudes of emotionally disturbed youth toward the elderly. *Educational Gerontology, 25*, 623–640.

Belgrave, M., & Darrow, A. A. (2010). The effect of participation in intergenerational music activities on participants' cross-age attitudes, positive nonverbal behaviors, and behaviors of engagement. In L. E. Schraer-Joiner (Ed.), *Proceedings of the 18th International Seminar of the Commission on Music in Special Education, Music Therapy, and Music Medicine.* Nedlands, WA: International Society for Music Education.

Bowers, J. (1998). Effects of an intergenerational choir for community-based seniors and college students on age-related attitudes. *Journal of Music Therapy, 35*, 2–18.

Corbin, D. E., Kagan, D. M., & Metal-Corbin, J. (1987). Content analysis of an intergenerational unit on aging in a sixth-grade classroom, *Educational Gerontology, 13*, 403–410.

Corbin, D. E., Metal-Corbin, J., & Barg, C. (1989). Teaching about aging in the elementary school: A one-year follow-up. *Educational Gerontology, 15*, 103–110.

Cote, N. G., Mosher-Ashley, P. M., & Kiernan, H. W. (2002). Linking long-term care residents with elementary students via a pen pal program. *Activities, Adaptation, & Aging, 27*(1), 1–11.

Cummings, S. M., Williams, M. M., & Ellis, R. A. (2002). Impact of an intergenerational program on 4th graders' attitudes toward elders and school behaviors. *Journal of Human Behavior in the Social Environment, 6*(3), 91–107.

Darrow, A. A., Johnson, C. M., & Ollenberger, T. (1994). The effect of participation in an intergenerational choir on teens' and older persons' cross-age attitudes. *Journal of Music Therapy, 31*, 119–134.

Dellmann-Jenkins, M., Fowler, L., Lambert, D. Fruit, D., & Richardson, R. (1994). Intergenerational sharing seminars: Their impact on young adult college students and senior guest students. *Educational Gerontology, 20*, 579–588.

Dellmann-Jenkins, M., Lambert, D., & Fruit, D. (1991). Fostering preschoolers' prosocial behaviors toward the elderly: The effect of an intergenerational program. *Educational Gerontology, 17*, 21–32.

Dunkle, R. E., & Mikelthun, B. G. (1983). Intergenerational programming: An adopt-a-grandparent program in a retirement community. *Activities, Adaptation, & Aging, 3*(2), 93–105.

Femia, E. E., Zarit, S. H., Blair, C., Jarrott, S. E., & Bruno, K. (2008). Intergenerational preschool experiences and the young child: Potential benefits to development. *Early Childhood Research Quarterly, 23*, 272–287.

Gamliel, T., Reichental, Y., & Eyal, N. (2007). Intergenerational educational encounters: Part 2: Counseling implications of the model. *Educational Gerontology, 33*, 145–164.

Giglio, L. L. (2006). *The effect of a music therapy intergenerational program on cued and spontaneous behaviors of older adults with dementia.* Unpublished master's thesis, University of Kansas.

Haber, E. A., & Short-DeGraff, M. A. (1990). Intergenerational programming for an increasingly age-segregated society. *Activities, Adaptation, & Aging, 14*(3), 35–49.

Hagestad, G. O., & Uhlenberg, P. (2006). Should we be concerned about age segregation? Some theoretical and empirical explorations. *Research on Aging, 28*(6), 638–653.

Hamilton, G., Brown, S., Alonzo, T., Glover, M., Mersereau, Y., & Wilson, P. (1998). Building community for the long term: An intergenerational commitment. *The Gerontologist, 39*, 235–238.

Herrmann, D. S., Sipsas-Herrmann, A., Stafford, M., & Herrmann, N. C. (2005). Benefits and risks of intergenerational program participation by senior citizens. *Educational Gerontology, 31*, 123–138.

Hill, H. (2007). Intergenerational dance/movement program in Melbourne, Australia. *Journal of Intergenerational Relationships, 5*(1), 97–101.

Jarrott, S. E., Gigliotti, C. M., & Smock, S. A. (2006). Where do we stand? Testing the foundation of a shared site intergenerational program. *Journal of Intergenerational Relationships, 4*(2), 73–92.

Kaplan, M., & Larkin, E. (2004). Launching intergenerational programs in early childhood settings: A comparison of explicit intervention with an emergent approach. *Early Childhood Education Journal, 31*(3), 157–163.

Karasik, R. J., & Wallingford, M. S. (2007). Finding community: Developing and maintaining effective intergenerational service-learning partnerships. *Educational Gerontology, 33*, 775–793.

Kassab, C., & Vance, L. (1999). An assessment of the effectiveness of an intergenerational program for youth. *Psychological Reports, 84*(1), 198–200.

Leitner, M. J. (1981). The effects of intergenerational music activities on senior day care participants and elementary school children. *Dissertation Abstracts International, 42*, 8A.

Lindquist, B. (1986). They need us, we need them: A study of the benefits of intergenerational contact. *Activities, Adaptation, & Aging, 8*(3/4), 83–94.

Lowenthal, B., & Egan, R. (1991). Senior citizen volunteers in a university day-care center. *Educational Gerontology, 17*, 363–378.

Lynott, P. P., & Merola, P. R. (2007). Improving the attitudes of 4th graders toward older people through a multidimensional intergeneration program. *Educational Gerontology, 33*, 64–74.

Marx, M. S., Hubbard, P., Cohen-Mansfield, J., Dakheel-Ali, M., & Thein, K. (2005). Community-service activities versus traditional activities in an intergenerational visiting program. *Educational Gerontology, 31*, 263–271.

Meshel, D. S., & McGlynn, R. P. (2004). Intergenerational contact, attitudes, and stereotypes of adolescents and older people. *Educational Gerontology, 30*, 457–479.

Middlecamp, M., & Gross, D. (2002). Intergenerational daycare and preschoolers' attitudes about aging. *Educational Gerontology, 28*, 271–288.

Newman, S., Karip, E., & Faux, R. B. (1995). Everyday memory function of older adults: The impact of intergenerational school volunteer programs. *Educational Gerontology, 21*, 569–580.

Newman, S., & Smith, T. B. (1997). Developmental theories as the basis for intergenerational programs. In C. Williams & K. Sheedy (Eds.), *Intergenerational programs: Past, present, and future* (pp. 3–19). Washington, DC: Taylor & Francis.

Newman, S., & Ward, C. (1992/1993). An observational study of intergenerational activities and behavior change in dementing elders at adult day care centers. *International Journal of Aging and Human Development, 36*(4), 321–333.

Peacock, J. R., & O'Quin, J. A. (2006). Higher education and foster grandparent programs: Exploring mutual benefits. *Educational Gerontology, 32*, 367–378.

Powell, J. A., & Arquitt, G. E. (1978). Getting the generations back together: A rationale for development of community based intergenerational interaction programs. *The Family Coordinator, 27*(4), 421–426.

Proller, N. L. (1989). The effects of an adoptive grandparent program on youth and elderly participants. *Journal of Children in Contemporary Society, 20*(3–4), 195–203.

Saltz, R. (1989). Research evaluation of a foster grandparent program. *Intergenerational Programs*, 205–217.

Saxon, S. V., & Etten, M. J. (2002). *Physical change and aging: A guide for the helping professions* (4th ed.). New York: Tiresias Press.

St. John, P. A. (2008). From swinging on a star to childhood chants: Infants and seniors create intergenerational counterpoint. In *Music in the early years: Research, theory and practice.*

Proceedings of the 13th International ISME Early Childhood Music Education Commission Seminar, Rome, Italy.

Stremmel, A. J., Travis, S. S., Kelly-Harrison, P., & Hensley, A. D. (1994). The perceived benefits and problems associated with intergenerational exchanges in day care settings. *The Gerontologist, 34*, 513–519.

Underwood, H. L., & Dorfman, L. T. (2006). A view from the other side: Elders' reactions to intergenerational service-learning. *Journal of Intergenerational Relationships, 4*(2), 43–60.

VanderVen, K. (1999). Intergenerational theory: The missing element in today's intergenerational programs. *Child & Youth Services, 20*(1/2), 33–47.

VanWeelden, K., & Whipple, J. (2004). Effect of field experiences on music therapy students' perceptions of choral music for geriatric wellness programs. *Journal of Music Therapy, 41*, 340–352.

Vernon, A. E. (1999). Designing for change: Attitudes toward the elderly and intergenerational programming. *Child & Youth Services, 20*(1/2), 161–173.

Ward, C. R., Kamp, L. L., & Newman, S. (1996). The effects of participation in an intergenerational program on the behavior of residents with dementia. *Activities, Adaptation, & Aging, 20*(4), 61–76.

White, E. M. (2001). Attitudes of preschool children toward the elderly at the Stride Rite Intergenerational Day Care Center. *Dissertation Abstracts International, 62*, 4A.

Whitehouse, P. J., & Whitehouse, C. C. (2005). The intergenerational school: Integrating intergenerational approaches in the care of those with age-related cognitive challenges. *Australasian Journal on Ageing, 24*, S57–S58.

Williams, A., & Nussbaum, J. F. (2001). *Intergenerational communication across the life span.* Mahwah, NJ: Lawrence Erlbaum Associates.

Zeldin, S., Larson, R., Camino, L., & O'Connor, C. (2005). Intergenerational relationships and partnerships in community programs: Purpose, practice, and directions for research. *Journal of Community Psychology, 33*(1), 1–10.

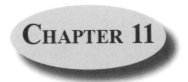

REVIEW OF THE RESEARCH LITERATURE ON INTERGENERATIONAL PROGRAMMING AND MUSIC THERAPY

My grand friends are very nice and hopefully they think that I'm fun. —John

Seeing their smiling faces every week gives me something to look forward to.
—Mr. W.

This chapter includes a review of literature pertaining to music-based intergenerational programs. Researchers who explore the benefits of music-based intergenerational programs have measured cross-age attitudes, cross-age interactions, and older adults' psychosocial well-being. The findings from the music-based intergenerational research studies are provided in this chapter and compared to the larger body of intergenerational research. Together this information will serve as the empirical framework for the next chapter, which provides music interventions for various healthcare professionals to employ when conducting music-based intergenerational programs.

MUSIC-BASED INTERGENERATIONAL PROGRAMS

Music participation, such as listening or singing to music, is an activity enjoyed by all age groups. Due to its appeal, it can serve as a vehicle to bridge the gap between generations. Music can be easily structured to facilitate inclusive practices with those who have different musical tastes and who represent different age groups. Research in music-based intergenerational programs has been conducted with older adults who live in residential facilities as well as those who reside in the community; and with younger participants including infants, elementary-age children, high school adolescents, and college-age young adults. Intergenerational choirs have been created that utilize the music of both generations, whereas other intergenerational groups have employed traditional music therapy interventions such as instrument playing, moving to music, singing, and academic and social skills training through music. Research in music-based intergenerational programs and in the larger body of intergenerational research has shared similar purposes. Researchers have examined the effect of intergenerational music groups on cross-age attitudes, cross-age interactions, and older adults' psychosocial well-being (Belgrave & Darrow, 2010; Bowers, 1998; Darrow, Johnson, & Ollenberger, 1994; Frego, 1995; St. John, 2008).

Intergenerational Performing Groups

Intergenerational performing groups have been created with younger and older persons in choral, orchestra, and band settings. These performing groups employ a learning-together intergenerational model where both generations learn new music together. The end result is usually an intergenerational concert in which the group performs the music literature that they have rehearsed. Frego (1995) discussed an intergenerational program titled Interlink, started by the Canadian Mental Health Association. Interlink is an intergenerational choir comprised of children and older adults. The structured program and choir has a curriculum based on the academic year that includes various methods for combining the two generations. The interactions are graduated, starting with the forming of pen-pal dyads consisting of younger and older persons. The younger and older choir members rehearse music in separate rehearsals. They then begin to meet together through structured social intergenerational activities and joint rehearsals. The culminating project for the academic year is a joint public performance, which usually includes a combined intergenerational choir as well as solos, duets, and songs performed by one generation. Conway and Hodgman (2008) combined an intact college choir and older adult community choir for a combined performance. Both choral groups participated in combined rehearsals in preparation for the concert. Participants from both generations shared that their musical experience helped to decrease the generation gap and, as a result, fostered mutual respect among all choral members, regardless of age.

Intergenerational orchestras are another type of music-based performing group. Lorraine Marks is the founder and director of two intergenerational orchestras: the New Jersey Intergenerational Choir and the Florida Intergenerational Orchestra of America ("Lorraine Marks' Orchestras Are for the Ages," 2009). The director shared that, in both of these programs, participation in the orchestra fostered intergenerational friendships between the younger and older persons. Additionally, the younger students were more willing to practice, and both generations participated in mutual teaching and learning. Alfano (2008) found similar benefits for both high school students and older adults who participated in an intergenerational band program in Canada. In this unique curriculum-based program, the intergenerational band meets at a high school during the school day. High school students enroll in the band as part of their high school curriculum, and older adult participants enroll in the intergenerational band through the high school as day students. Christopher Alfano, the director, found that participation in the group has created cross-age mentoring relationships as well as mutual learners, as high school students and older adults learn new music together. Other music-based intergenerational programs have been examined more closely by researchers to determine the specific benefits afforded to younger and older participants.

CROSS-AGE ATTITUDES

Attitudes are comprised of three components—feelings, knowledge, and behaviors. The feeling component of an attitude is based on an individual's emotion toward another person. The knowledge component pertains to an individual's knowledge and understanding about another person. The behavior component is developed based on the interactions that an individual has with another person (Lemme, 2002; Williams & Nussbaum, 2001). Many intergenerational programs have been created to improve cross-age attitudes between children and older adults. Negative cross-age attitudes are composed of stereotypes directed to the other generation and are often the result of decreased interaction between younger and older generations. The attitudinal focus of intergenerational research has been driven by findings from Rich, Myrick, and Campbell (1983), who identified that aging attitudes begin to form as early as age 3. Changes in cross-age attitudes have been measured before and after intergenerational activities through formal measures, such as standardized assessments; and through informal measures, such as researcher-developed questionnaires, structured interviews, and focus groups (Corbin, Kagan, & Metal-Corbin, 1987; Corbin, Metal-Corbin, & Barg, 1989; Femia, Zarit, Blair, Jarrott, & Bruno, 2008; Lynott & Merola, 2007; Marks, Newman, & Onawola, 1985; Middlecamp & Gross, 2002; Proller, 1989; Schwalbach & Kiernan, 2002; Seefeldt, 1987; White, 2001).

The research literature exploring older adults' attitudes toward younger persons is limited, and there is often little use of standardized instruments. Intergenerational programs exploring older persons' attitudes toward younger generations have been conducted with community-dwelling older adults, older persons living in nursing homes and independent and assisted living facilities, and individuals attending adult daycare programs. The younger generation has consisted of preschoolers, elementary-age children, adolescents, and young adults. Findings from the research literature have shown an improvement in older adults' attitudes toward preschoolers, elementary-age children, adolescents, and young adults after participation in intergenerational programs. Additionally, older adults have reported that they understood and could better relate to familial and non-familial younger persons (Dellmann-Jenkins, Fowler, Lambert, Fruit, & Richardson, 1994; DeSouza, 2007; Jones, Herrick, & York, 2004; Underwood & Dorfman, 2006).

Many intergenerational studies have focused on changing younger generations' attitudes toward older adults. The younger generation in these studies has included preschoolers, elementary-age children, adolescents, and young adults. The older generation has included community-dwelling well-elderly and older adults attending adult daycare programs, intergenerational daycare programs, and older persons residing in nursing homes and continuous care retirement centers. Changes in young persons' attitudes have been measured before and after intergenerational activities through formal and informal measures. Results of attitudinal research toward aging have been mixed for the younger generations. Some researchers found that attitudes toward aging moved from negative to positive after intergenerational interactions, while others reported that younger persons' views did not change or became negative (Aday, Aday, Arnold, & Bendix, 1996; Corbin et al., 1989; Femia et al., 2008; Ferraro, 1997; Kassab & Vance, 1999; Middlecamp & Gross, 2002; Newman, Lyons, & Onawola, 1985; O'Hanlon & Brookover, 2002; Schwalbach & Kiernan, 2002; Seefeldt, 1987; White, 2001).

Cross-Age Attitudes and Music-Based Intergenerational Programs

Several researchers have examined the effect of participation in a music-based intergenerational program on cross-age attitudes (Belgrave & Darrow, 2010; Bowers, 1998; Darrow et al., 1994; Leitner, 1981). Leitner (1981) conducted a study with elementary-age children and older adults who participated in a recreational music-based intergenerational program. Children interacted with older adults who attended an adult daycare facility for six weekly sessions. Activities in the intergenerational sessions included singing, instrument playing, and music games. A researcher-developed assessment was used to measure cross-age attitudes of older adults and children. Older adults' attitudes toward children became more positive for older persons who participated in the intergenerational program compared to older individuals who did not have intergenerational contact, but this increase did not reach significance. Results also showed that children's attitudes toward older adults improved after the intergenerational program.

Researchers have also employed younger and older generations learning-together models to create intergenerational choirs. An early study conducted by Darrow et al. (1994) combined older adults and high-school adolescents in an intergenerational choir. Community-dwelling older adults and high school students joined an intergenerational choir, which met for weekly rehearsals throughout the fall and spring semesters. Additionally, the older adults and high school students participated in various social activities and gave 22 performances throughout the two semesters. The repertoire for the choir included music that was familiar to both generations, such as patriotic songs and show tunes, as well as the preferred music of each generation, which may have been unfamiliar to the other generation. During the rehearsals, the high school students were interspersed among the older adults. Cross-age attitudes were measured using the Age Group Evaluation and Description (AGED) Inventory (Knox, Gekoski, & Kelly, 1995). This attitudinal measure contains 28 pairs of bipolar adjectives rated on a 7-point Likert-type scale. The assessment consists of four subscales, two of which are evaluative—goodness and positiveness, and two of which are descriptive—vitality and maturity. Results showed that older male participants' attitudes toward teen males became more positive on the goodness and maturity subscales. Older male and female participants' attitudes toward teen females also became more positive, but did not reach significance. Results also showed that the high school students' attitudes toward older males and females improved after participation in the intergenerational choir. Additionally, high school students' attitudes toward older adult males showed more improvement than attitudes toward older females.

Bowers (1998) conducted a similar study with an intergenerational choir comprised of college-age young adults and community-dwelling older adults. College students from a women's glee club participated in a two-semester Adopt-A-Choir program, and a local senior choir served as the adopted choir. The intergenerational choir gave two performances, one each semester. The weekly rehearsals included singing and structured activities such as conversations and games. The structured activities were utilized to foster positive interactions between the two generations. Repertoire for the intergenerational choir included music that was familiar to each generation. Big Band music was selected as familiar music to older adults and contemporary gospel music was selected as familiar music to the college-age students. Cross-age attitudes were measured using the AGED inventory (Knox et al., 1995). Results showed that older adult participants' attitudes toward young adults improved after their involvement in the intergenerational choir. Similarly, college-age young adults' attitudes toward older adults improved after participation in the intergenerational choir.

Bales, Eklund, and Siffin (2000) combined fourth graders and older adults from the community in an intergenerational choir. Children were asked to identify three words to describe older adults. These words were then categorized as positive, negative, physical descriptor, or other. Children and older adults were assigned a cross-age pen pal and exchanged letters for 8 weeks prior to the intergenerational choir program. The intergenerational choir rehearsals occurred weekly for a month. Rehearsals included structured activities and conversations followed by singing. Results showed that children's descriptions of older adults contained an increase in the number of positive words and a decrease in the number of negative words used to describe older adults after their participation in an intergenerational choir.

Researchers employing learning-together music-based intergenerational programs have also utilized traditional music therapy interventions to improve cross-age attitudes between children and older adults. Music therapy interventions include singing, moving to music, instrument playing, songwriting, and structured conversations. During these sessions, younger persons were interspersed among the older participants. Some interventions, such as group singing and instrument playing, occurred in a large group setting, whereas other activities, such as structured conversation and moving to music, occurred between younger and older person dyads. Singing activities included songs that were familiar and unfamiliar to both age groups. Instrument-playing activities required children and older participants to play simple melodic and rhythmic accompaniment patterns to familiar and newly learned songs. Songs from the singing intervention were selected based on themes that engaged both generations. These themes were then used to stimulate conversations between children and older participants.

Belgrave and Darrow (2010) employed this model to examine cross-age attitudes of older adults and children. Older adult participants from an independent and assisted-living facility interacted with elementary-age children in a 6-week intergenerational program. Older adults' attitudes toward children were measured using the AGED inventory (Knox et al., 1995). Children's attitudes toward older adults were measured through the AGED inventory, as well as a written paragraph titled "What It's Like to Be Old." Results showed that older adults' attitudes toward young boys became more positive in respect to maturity. However, older adults' attitudes toward young girls did not change. Results of the formal and informal measures showed positive and negative changes in children's attitudes. Children's attitudes toward older women did not change after the intergenerational interactions. Children's attitudes toward older males varied, depending on the specific subscale. Children rated older males higher in vitality after the intergenerational program, but rated older males lower in goodness and maturity after the intergenerational program. The paragraphs were analyzed for positive and negative words and themes. Results showed a decrease in the amount of negative words used to describe older adults. Also, the ratio of positive and negative themes in the paragraphs changed after children's participation in the intergenerational program. Before the intergenerational program, children identified more negative than positive themes to describe older adults. On the posttest paragraph, children identified more positive than negative themes to describe the older adults.

Belgrave (2009) used a similar model in a 10-week intergenerational program. The researcher employed the Children's Attitudes Toward the Elderly (CATE; Jantz, Seefeldt, Galper, & Serock, 1980), the AGED inventory (Knox et al., 1995), and biweekly open-ended questionnaires to measure changes in cross-age attitudes. Results of standardized and informal attitudinal measures were mixed. Standardized measures revealed that children's attitudes toward older adults improved after interacting with older adults, although not significantly so. Results of biweekly post-session questionnaires revealed a decrease in negative descriptions of older adults and an increase in positive descriptions of older adults, suggesting a more positive view toward aging. Results revealed that older adults' attitudes toward children improved significantly after their participation in the intergenerational program.

Not all empirical studies pertaining to cross-age attitudes have measured the attitudes of the younger and older generations participating in the intergenerational program. Some music researchers have examined cross-age attitudes for individuals who observed an intergenerational performance. Darrow, Johnson, Ollenberger, and Miller (2001) examined cross-age attitudes of high school students and older adults before and after attending an intergenerational choir concert. Results of the AGED inventory (Knox et al., 1995) revealed an improvement in cross-age attitudes of teenagers and older adults after attending the intergenerational choir concert.

Factors that Influence the Younger Generation's Attitudes toward Older Adults

There are five factors that may contribute to the mixed results of younger persons' attitudes toward aging: functioning level of the older adults, length of the intergenerational program, differences in attitudinal measures, younger persons' attitudes toward aging prior to intergenerational contact, and the multidimensionality of the younger generation's attitudes. The physical and cognitive declines associated with some age-related illnesses affect older adults' level of engagement in intergenerational sessions. Some researchers found that when older adults were unable to participate in many of the activities due to their severe declines, children held more negative attitudes toward aging (Barton, 1999; Seefeldt, 1987). The length of the intergenerational program also may have contributed to mixed results. Many of the intergenerational studies lasted for several weeks, months, or an academic calendar year. However, there were two studies in the literature in which the intergenerational programs lasted for 1 week or less (Corbin et al., 1987; Couper, Sheehan, & Thomas, 1991). It may be an unrealistic expectation that younger persons involved in a short intergenerational program would quickly change their attitude toward aging in a positive direction.

Inconsistencies in attitudinal measures may affect the mixed findings for younger persons' attitudes toward the process of aging. Measuring attitudes is complex because attitudes are comprised of three components: feelings, knowledge, and behaviors. Some attitudinal measures examine all three components of the younger person's attitude, whereas other measures examine only one or two components. Attitudinal measures also differ in their definition of attitude. Several measures examine the three components of attitude, yet other attitudinal measures assess only stereotypes, personality traits, an individual's knowledge of aging, or social acceptance of an older adult—defined as how willing someone is to interact in a social setting with an older person. Therefore, direct comparisons between studies utilizing such various measures is difficult and thus is another factor that may contribute to mixed findings among younger generations' attitudes toward older adults. It is important to use an assessment that measures all three components of attitudes to assess how intergenerational programs may affect aging (Vernon, 1999).

Sometimes both the younger and the older generation already hold a positive view toward the other generation. If this is true, then it is difficult to detect a significant improvement in their attitudes due to the ceiling effect. Finally, some researchers contribute the mixed findings to the belief that children's attitudes toward older adults are multidimensional, not one-dimensional (Mitchell, Wilson, Revicki, & Parker, 1985; Seefeldt 1987). Some aspects of aging may be identified as positive, but other aspects (e.g., physical or psychological declines) may be identified as negative. Perhaps it is unrealistic to expect the younger generation to not be aware of or to not be alarmed by the natural physical or cognitive declines that occur with the aging process. Some studies have shown that although children may identify those parts of aging as negative, it does not change or influence their willingness to interact with older adults. Some adolescents even continued their intergenerational interactions after the program finished.

CROSS-AGE INTERACTIONS

A secondary focus of research conducted in the area of intergenerational programming has been the improvement of cross-age interactions. Several researchers have investigated the type and frequency of intergenerational interactions between younger and older generations through the use of social acceptance measures and behavioral observations. Researchers have been particularly interested in children and young adults' willingness to share, cooperate, and interact with older adults. Researchers have also observed interaction behaviors and levels of engagement exhibited by both younger and older generations participating in intergenerational programs. The results of many of these investigations indicated that younger and older persons' cross-age interactions improved as a result of their participation in intergenerational programs (Angersbach & Jones-Forster, 1999; Ferraro, 1997; Hamilton et al., 1998; Kuehne, 1992; Newman, Morris, & Streetman, 1999; O'Rourke, 1999).

Various measures have been used to examine prosocial behaviors, social acceptance, and social distance in intergenerational studies involving preschoolers, elementary-age children, and young adults. *Prosocial behaviors* are defined as an individual's willingness to share, help, and cooperate with another person. *Social acceptance* is an individual's ability to accept and interact with another person who is different. *Social distance* is an individual's level of comfort in interacting with another person in varying degrees of closeness. Studies have shown that children and young adults participating in intergenerational programs have reported that they feel more comfortable interacting and communicating with older adults after participating in an intergenerational program. Behavioral observations of cross-age interactions revealed that positive cross-age interactions occur more frequently than negative cross-age interactions during structured intergenerational activities. Additionally, older adults participating in intergenerational activities have exhibited more engagement behaviors than when they engage in activities without younger persons present (Dellman-Jenkins, Lambert, & Fruit, 1991; Dellmann-Jenkins et al., 1994; Femia et al., 2008; Ferraro, 1997; Hamilton et al., 1998; O'Rourke, 1999; Short-DeGraff & Diamond, 1996).

Cross-Age Interactions and Music-Based Intergenerational Programs

Cross-age interactions have been measured through the younger generations' comfort and willingness to interact with older adults and through behavior observation of intergenerational interactions. Three of the studies described earlier in the cross-age attitudes section also examined children's interactions with older adults during music-based intergenerational programs. Bales et al. (2000) required children to keep a weekly journal to record their experiences during the intergenerational program. A content analysis was done on the journals to identify common themes in regard to the cross-age interactions. Qualitative data obtained from student journals resulted in four common themes: (1) the children realized that they had many things in common with the older adults, (2) the children perceived that they had developed a friendship with the older adults, (3) the children felt disappointed when the older adults left and they looked forward to the next meeting, and (4) the children expressed their desire to maintain contact with the older adults upon completion of the program.

Belgrave and Darrow (2010) measured children's comfort and willingness to interact with older adult participants during the structured conversations. Children wrote down in a notebook the responses that occurred with the older adults during the structured conversations. A frequency count was conducted on the weekly responses. Results showed a steady increase in the number of responses identified each week that indicated an increased comfort for the children when interacting with older adults.

Belgrave (2009) examined seven cross-age interaction behaviors between children and older adults during four interventions: singing, structured conversation, moving to music, and instrument playing. The seven interaction behaviors were on-task participation, smiles, touches, looks, encourages, assists partner, and initiates conversation with partner. Results of behavior observations indicated there was a difference in the type and frequency of interactions that occurred between children and older adults during singing, structured conversation, moving to music, and instrument-playing interventions. Structured conversation and moving to music elicited more interaction behaviors than singing and instrument playing for child and older adult participants. The intervention of singing also elicited more interaction behaviors for children than instrument playing. Interaction behaviors that occurred at a high frequency for child participants were "looks at older adult," "smiles," and "initiates conversation with older adult." Similarly, "smiles," "looks at child," and "initiates conversation with child" were interaction behaviors that occurred most frequently for older adult participants. "Initiates conversation with older adult," "encourages child," or "assists child" were interaction behaviors that occurred less frequently for both child and older adult participants.

VanWeelden and Whipple (2004) also combined college students and older adults in an intergenerational choir. College music therapy students interacted with an older adult choir for a semester practicum. The senior choir, comprised of older adults from the community, met weekly for a semester, concluding with an intergenerational concert. In this study, students served as conductors and performers. Students conducted one song during the rehearsals and participated as a choir member. Students' willingness and comfort with cross-age interactions were measured through a researcher-created assessment. The assessment consisted of 14 questions rated on a 7-point Likert-type scale. The assessment measured college students' comfort in interacting with older adults, perception of older adult singers in a choir, perception of older adults as learners in a choir, and willingness to lead an older adult choir in the future. The results showed that college students were more comfortable working with older adults in a choir after the intergenerational choir program. College students perceived that older adults were able to participate and function as a choir member, and thus were willing to conduct an older adult choir in the future as a result of participation in the project.

St. John (2008) conducted a unique study that examined cross-age interactions through observations and older adults' self-report. This study combined multiple generations, infants, caregivers, and older adults in a music-based program. Ages of the infants ranged from 3 to 16 months, and retired nuns volunteered to serve as older adult participants. The multiple generations participated in music activities such as singing, instrument playing, and moving to music. Older adults' experiences were examined through their weekly journal entries and observation of cross-age interactions during the music activities. Results of journal entries revealed that older adults initially felt anxious and hesitant about interacting with infants. These feelings decreased as the program continued and resulted in the older adults' increased comfort in interacting with the infants. Direct observations of infants during the music program showed that infants began to initiate interactions with older adults during the music activities.

Three additional studies used behavior observations to measure older adults' experiences and cross-age interactions during intergenerational music programs. These studies examined the interactions between preschool-age children and older adults who had dementia. Newman and Ward (1992/1993) observed positive verbal and nonverbal behaviors of older adults who had dementia. The nine behaviors examined were smiling, extending hands, clapping hands, tapping feet, singing, verbal interaction, touching, hugging, and nodding head. The results revealed that touching and extending hands occurred more during the intergenerational sessions than when children were not present. Similar results were found in a follow-up study conducted by Ward, Kamp, and Newman (1996), who found that older adults exhibited more touching during intergenerational music programs than music activities without children. In a more recent study, Giglio (2006) also examined the change in behaviors of older adults when children were present during music therapy groups. Findings for this study were similar; older adults exhibited more spontaneous behaviors when interacting with children during intergenerational sessions. Older adults were also more alert and oriented to their environment when children were present. The studies described here support the benefits both generations receive from participating in intergenerational programs. However, as stated earlier, the majority of intergenerational research has focused on the benefits afforded to the younger generation. As the field continues to grow, more research needs to be conducted to examine the additional benefits received by older adults as a result of their participation in intergenerational programs.

PSYCHOSOCIAL WELL-BEING

During the aging process, older adults may experience isolation from their family, friends, and society. An older person's role as caretaker for their family may begin to diminish as they age, resulting in a perception that they are not needed by their adult children. Additionally, age-related declines may cause older adults to move closer to their children or into senior living communities, which may contribute to their disconnection from their long-term friends and society. These changes in living conditions, roles, and health for older persons can result in decreased feelings of usefulness and purpose in life and may affect their overall psychosocial well-being. Psychosocial well-being is a subjective measure affected by many factors, including but not limited to change in family structure, change in living conditions, and change in cognitive and physical functioning. Measures of psychosocial well-being have examined individuals' satisfaction with life, sense of purpose, feelings of usefulness, and contributions to other generations and society. Intergenerational programs have provided opportunities for older adults to reconnect to society through participation in meaningful activities, which enhances feelings of usefulness. Older adults who participated in intergenerational programs have cited feelings of helpfulness, usefulness, happiness, decreased isolation, improved self-esteem, and life satisfaction as perceived benefits resulting from their intergenerational interactions (Dellmann-Jenkins et al., 1994; Marx, Hubbard, Cohen-Mansfield, Dakheel-Ali, & Thein, 2005; Proller, 1989; Schirm, Ross-Alaolmolki, & Conrad, 1995; White, 2008).

Psychosocial Well-Being and Music-Based Intergenerational Programs

Researchers conducting studies in intergenerational programs have begun to focus on the benefits received by older adults. One area of focus that is growing is older adults' psychosocial well-being. Many studies have begun to explore the relationship between older adults' participation in intergenerational programs and their well-being. A few studies have examined the effect of participation in a music-based intergenerational program on older adults' well-being. Leitner (1981) examined older adults' psychological well-being and life satisfaction with the Affect Balance Scale (Bradburn, 1963). The scale consists of 10 close-ended questions, 5 of which are positive and 5 that are negative. Life satisfaction was measured by one question on a 5-point Likert-type scale. Results showed that older adults in the intergenerational music group did not have improved well-being or life satisfaction when compared to older adults who did not have intergenerational contact. However, results should be interpreted cautiously as the Affect Balance Scale has low reliability as reported by Schulz, Obrien, and Tompkins (as cited in Coffman, 2002). Belgrave (2009) examined older adults' psychosocial well-being through measuring their perceived feelings of usefulness after weekly music-based intergenerational sessions. Older adults rated their perception of usefulness to others on a 7-point Likert-type scale. Results revealed that older adults perceived a weekly increase in their feelings of usefulness after participating in a music-based intergenerational program.

There are only a few music-based studies that have been conducted to examine older adults' psychosocial well-being. Additionally, psychosocial well-being is a broad category that is influenced by many factors. It is important for music researchers to continue to explore ways in which participation in music-based intergenerational programs affects various aspects of psychosocial well-being. The type of intergenerational program, the role of the older adult during the intergenerational program, and how useful the older adult feels all influence an older person's perceived well-being. Interviewing older adults after their participation in intergenerational programs is a useful approach to understanding how older adults perceive these programs and how these programs affect their overall psychosocial well-being.

REFERENCES

Aday, R. H., Aday, K. L., Arnold, J. L., & Bendix, S. L. (1996). Changing children's perceptions of the elderly: The effects of intergenerational contact. *Gerontology & Geriatrics Education, 16*(3), 37–51.

Alfano, C. J. (2008). Intergenerational learning in a high school environment. *International Journal of Community Music, 1*(2), 253–267.

Angersbach, H. L., & Jones-Forster, S. (1999). Intergenerational interactions: A descriptive analysis of elder-child interactions in a campus-based child care center. *Child & Youth Services, 20*(1/2), 117–128.

Bales, S. S., Eklund, S. J., & Siffin, C. F. (2000). Children's perceptions of elders before and after a school-based intergenerational program. *Educational Gerontology, 26*, 677–689.

Belgrave, M. (2009). *The effect of a music-based intergenerational program on children and older adults' intergenerational interactions, cross-age attitudes, and older adults' psychosocial well-being.* Unpublished doctoral dissertation, Florida State University.

Belgrave, M., & Darrow, A. A. (2010). The effect of participation in intergenerational music activities on participants' cross-age attitudes, positive nonverbal behaviors, and behaviors of engagement. In L. E. Schraer-Joiner (Ed.), *Proceedings of the 18th International Seminar of the Commission on Music in Special Education, Music Therapy, and Music Medicine.* Nedlands, WA: International Society for Music Education.

Bowers, J. (1998). Effects of an intergenerational choir for community-based seniors and college students on age-related attitudes. *Journal of Music Therapy, 35*, 2–18.

Bradburn, N. M., & Noll, E. (1969). *The structure of psychological well-being.* Chicago: Aldine.

Coffman, D. D. (2002). Music and quality of life in older adults. *Psychomusicology, 18*(1–2), 76–88.

Conway, C., & Hodgman, T. M. (2008). College and community choir member experiences in a collaborative intergenerational performance project. *Journal of Research in Music Education, 56*(3), 220–238.

Corbin, D. E., Kagan, D. M., & Metal-Corbin, J. (1987). Content analysis of an intergenerational unit on aging in a sixth-grade classroom. *Educational Gerontology, 13*, 403–410.

Corbin, D. E., Metal-Corbin, J., & Barg, C. (1989). Teaching about aging in the elementary school: A one-year follow-up. *Educational Gerontology, 15*, 103–110.

Couper, D. P., Sheehan, N. W., & Thomas, E. L. (1991). Attitude toward old people: The impact of an intergenerational program. *Educational Gerontology, 17*, 41–53.

Darrow, A. A., Johnson, C. M., & Ollenberger, T. (1994). The effect of participation in an intergenerational choir on teens' and older persons' cross-age attitudes. *Journal of Music Therapy, 31*, 119–134.

Darrow, A. A., Johnson, C., Ollenberger, T., & Miller, A. M. (2001). The effect of an intergenerational choir performance on audience members' attitudinal statements toward teens and older persons. *International Journal of Music Education, Original Series, 38*(1), 43–50.

Dellmann-Jenkins, M., Lambert, D., & Fruit, D. (1991). Fostering preschoolers' prosocial behaviors toward the elderly: The effect of an intergenerational program. *Educational Gerontology, 17*, 21–32.

Dellman-Jenkins, M., Fowler, L., Lambert, D., Fruit, D., & Richardson, R. (1994). Intergenerational sharing seminars: Their impact on young adult college students and senior guest students. *Educational Gerontology, 20*, 579–588.

Femia, E. E., Zarit, S. H., Blair, C., Jarrott, S. E., & Bruno, K. (2008). Intergenerational preschool experiences and the young child: Potential benefits to development. *Early Childhood Research Quarterly, 23*, 272–287.

Ferraro, C. A. (1997). *The effect of intergenerational activities on the attitudes, feelings, and behaviors of cognitively impaired older adults.* Unpublished master's thesis, University of Southern California.

Frego, R. J. D. (1995). Uniting the generations with music programs. *Music Educators Journal, 81*(6), 17–19.

Gamliel, T., Reichental, Y., & Eyal, N. (2007). Intergenerational educational encounters: Part 2: Counseling implications of the model. *Educational Gerontology, 33*, 145–164.

Giglio, L. L. (2006). *The effect of a music therapy intergenerational program on cued and spontaneous behaviors of older adults with dementia.* Unpublished master's thesis, University of Kansas.

Hamilton, G., Brown, S., Alonzo, T., Glover, M., Mersereau, Y., & Wilson, P. (1998). Building community for the long term: An intergenerational commitment. *The Gerontologist, 39*, 235–238.

Herrmann, D. S., Sipsas-Herrmann, A., Stafford, M., & Herrmann, N. C. (2005). Benefits and risks of intergenerational program participation by senior citizens. *Educational Gerontology, 31*, 123–138.

Jantz, R., Seefeldt, C., Galper, A., & Serock, K. (1976). *Test manual: The CATE, Children's Attitudes Toward the Elderly.* College Park, MA: University of Maryland, Center on Aging and the University of Maryland, College of Education.

Jones, E. D., Herrick, C., & York, R. F. (2004). An intergenerational group benefits both emotionally disturbed youth and older adults. *Issues in Mental Health Nursing, 25*(8), 753–767.

Karasik, R. J., & Wallingford, M. S. (2007). Finding community: Developing and maintaining effective intergenerational service-learning partnerships. *Educational Gerontology, 33*, 775–793.

Kassab, C., & Vance, L. (1999). An assessment of the effectiveness of an intergenerational program for youth. *Psychological Reports, 84*(1), 198–200.

Knox, V. J., Gekoski, W. L., & Kelly, L. E. (1995). The Age Group Evaluation and Description (AGED) Inventory: A new instrument for assessing stereotypes of and attitudes toward age groups. *International Journal for Aging and Human Development, 40*, 31–55.

Kuehne, V. S. (1992). Older adults in intergenerational programs: What are their experiences really like? *Activities, Adaptation, & Aging, 16*(4), 49–67.

Leitner, M. J. (1981). The effects of intergenerational music activities on senior day care participants and elementary school children. *Dissertation Abstracts International, 42*, 8A.

Lemme, B. H. (2002). *Development in adulthood.* Needham Heights, MA: Allyn & Bacon.

Lorraine Marks' orchestras are for the ages. (2009). *International Musician, 107*(10), 28.

Lynott, P. P., & Merola, P. R. (2007). Improving the attitudes of 4th graders toward older people through a multidimensional intergeneration program. *Educational Gerontology, 33*, 64–74.

Marks, R., Newman, S., & Onawola, R. (1985). Latency-aged children's views of aging. *Educational Gerontology, 11*, 89–99.

Marx, M. S., Hubbard, P., Cohen-Mansfield, J., Dakheel-Ali, M., & Thein, K. (2005). Community-service activities versus traditional activities in an intergenerational visiting program. *Educational Gerontology, 31*, 263–271.

Middlecamp, M., & Gross, D. (2002). Intergenerational daycare and preschoolers' attitudes about aging. *Educational Gerontology, 28*, 271–288.

Mitchell, J., Wilson, K., Revicki, D., & Parker, L. (1985). Children's perceptions of aging: A multidimensional approach to differences by age, sex, and race. *The Gerontologist, 25*, 182–187.

Newman, S., Lyons, C. W., & Onawola, R. S. T. (1985). The development of an intergenerational service-learning program at a nursing home. *The Gerontologist, 25*, 130–133.

Newman, S., Morris, G. A., & Streetman, H. (1999). Elder-child interaction analysis: An observation instrument for classrooms involving older adults as mentors, tutors, or resource persons. *Child & Youth Services, 20*(1/2), 129–145.

Newman, S., & Ward, C. (1992–1993). An observational study of intergenerational activities and behavior change in dementing elders at adult day care centers. *International Journal of Aging and Human Development, 36*(4), 321–333.

O'Hanlon, A. M., & Brookover, B. C. (2002). Assessing changes in attitudes about aging: Personal reflections and a standardized measure. *Educational Gerontology, 28*, 711–725.

O'Rourke, K. A. (1999). Intergenerational programming: Yesterday's memories, today's moments, and tomorrow's hopes. *Dissertation Abstracts International, 61*, 1A.

Proller, N. L. (1989). The effects of an adoptive grandparent program on youth and elderly participants. *Journal of Children in Contemporary Society, 20*(3–4), 195–203.

Rich, P. E., Myrick, R. D., & Campbell, C. (1983). Changing children's perceptions of the elderly. *Educational Gerontology, 9*, 483–491.

Schirm, V., Ross-Alaolmolki, K. & Conrad, M. (1995). Collaborative education through a foster grandparent program: Enhancing intergenerational relations. *Gerontology & Geriatrics Education, 15*(3), 85–94.

Schwalbach, E., & Kiernan, S. (2002). Effects of an intergenerational friendly visit program on the attitudes of fourth graders toward elders. *Educational Gerontology, 28*, 175–187.

Seefeldt, C. (1987). The effects of preschoolers' visits to a nursing home. *The Gerontologist, 27*, 228–232.

Short-DeGraff, M. A., & Diamond, K. (1996). Intergenerational program effects on social responses of elderly adult day care members. *Educational Gerontology, 22*, 467–482.

St. John, P. A. (2008). *From swinging on a star to childhood chants: Infants and seniors create intergenerational counterpoint.* Proceedings of the 13th International ISME Early Childhood Music Education Commission Seminar, Rome, Italy.

Underwood, H. L., & Dorfman, L. T. (2006). A view from the other side: Elders' reactions to intergenerational service-learning. *Journal of Intergenerational Relationships, 4*(2), 43– 60.

VanWeelden, K., & Whipple, J. (2004). Effect of field experiences on music therapy students' perceptions of choral music for geriatric wellness programs. *Journal of Music Therapy, 41*, 340–352.

Vernon, A. E. (1999). Designing for change: Attitudes toward the elderly and intergenerational programming. *Child & Youth Services, 20*(1/2), 161–173.

Ward, C. R., Kamp, L. L., & Newman, S. (1996). The effects of participation in an intergenerational program on the behavior of residents with dementia. *Activities, Adaptation, & Aging, 20*(4), 61–76.

White, E. M. (2001). Attitudes of preschool children toward the elderly at the stride rite intergenerational day care center. *Dissertation Abstracts International, 62*, 4A.

Williams, A., & Nussbaum, J. F. (2001). *Intergenerational communication across the life span.* Mahwah, NJ: Lawrence Erlbaum Associates.

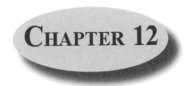

CHAPTER 12

CLINICAL APPLICATIONS FOR INTERGENERATIONAL PROGRAMMING

I've enjoyed playing music and singing songs with my grand friends. —Julie

I was able to share knowledge that I have learned through life experiences during the intergenerational program. —Mrs. C.

This chapter contains clinical applications that can be employed when working with music-based intergenerational programs. The chapter is divided into four focus areas that correspond to the four models of intergenerational programs: (1) employing music in an older generation serving younger generation model, (2) employing music in a younger generation serving older generation model, (3) employing music in a younger generation and older generation learning-together model, and (4) employing music in a younger generation and older generation recreational model. Each focus area is divided into clinical applications for general staff, volunteer musicians, and music therapists. The clinical applications also contain target behaviors for each generation, a guide to music selection for the intervention, advanced preparation required, and implementation directions.

FOCUS AREA 1: EMPLOYING MUSIC IN AN OLDER GENERATION SERVING YOUNGER GENERATION MODEL

Clinical Application 4.1 —————————————————————

Target Behavior–Younger Generation: Improve academic skills (letter and word recognition)

Target Behavior–Older Generation: Provide an opportunity to serve as a mentor for young children

Music: Choose music from a variety of familiar and simple children's songs that contain repetitive letter sounds. This type of music is often found in sections of stores and websites that pertain to academic learning skills for children.

Level 1—General Staff

Activity Name: "Learning Letters"

Advanced Preparation: Identify children's songs that contain a high level of repetition for one letter sound. For example, the songs "Baby Beluga" and "Brown Bear, Brown Bear, What Do You See?" have a high level of repetition for the letter "B." Once songs are identified, locate audio recordings for use in the intergenerational activity. Some children's songs have board books that contain an illustrated version of the song. If unable to locate a board book or if one does not exist for the song, one can be created by using clip art or a similar program to create pictures that relate to the lyrics and start with the specific letter. In addition, create large cutouts of the letter that will be used for the activity. For the songs discussed above, large cutouts of the letter "B" are created. Create enough letters for each older adult participant to hold.

Activity Direction: Introduce the song to the intergenerational group by playing the audio recording of the song while following along with the board book. Announce to the group that they will sing songs about a specific letter. Pass out large cutouts of letters to older adult participants and explain that they will point to or hold up the large letter whenever that sound is sung during the song. Play the audio recording again and encourage the participants to sing while the older adult participants point to or hold up the letter.

Level 2—Volunteer Musician

Activity Name: "Learning Letters"

Advanced Preparation: Learn the words and accompaniment to children's songs that have a high repetition for one letter sound. For example, the song "My Bonnie Lies over the Ocean," has a high level of repetition for the letter "B." Another simple and familiar song, "Old McDonald Had a Farm," can be used by selecting animals that all start with the same letter. For example, animals such as cat, cow, and calf can be selected for the letter "C." Create picture or letter manipulatives for the older adult participants to hold. To create picture manipulatives, locate images of items that start with the specific letter. For example, a picture of a cat may be used when working on the letter "C" during "Old McDonald Had a Farm." To create letter manipulatives, make large cutouts of specific letters to accompany song. For example, large cutouts of the letter "B" would be created when working on the letter "B" in "My Bonnie Lies over the Ocean." Create enough manipulatives for all of the older adult participants in the intergenerational group.

Activity Direction: Introduce the song to the intergenerational group by singing while playing an accompaniment instrument. Once the group is familiar with the song, explain that the children will learn a specific letter. Pass out the picture manipulatives to the older adult participants. Sing the song again with the older adult participants pointing to or holding up the picture. Pass out the letter manipulatives to the older adult participants. Sing the song once more and have the older adult participants point to the letter.

Level 3—Board-Certified Music Therapist

Activity Name: "Learning Words"

Other Goals Addressed–Younger Generation: Improve Positive Attitude toward Aging, Increase Children's Level of Comfort Interacting with Older Adults

Other Goals Addressed–Older Generation: Increase Meaningful Interactions, Increase Feelings of Usefulness, Increase Feelings of Generativity (Generativity is a measure of psychosocial well-being defined by Erik Erikson as a desire in adults to be concerned with or to contribute something to a younger generation.)

Advanced Preparation: Work with the classroom teacher to identify 2-letter, 3-letter, and 4-letter words that child participants have not learned. A good resource to determine appropriate words is the Dolch Sight Word list. The list consists of words that children should recognize by sight and is categorized by a child's grade in school. The lists are created for children from pre-kindergarten to third grade. Once the words are identified, choose a preexisting song or create a simple melody to teach the spelling of the words. For example, the 3-letter word *red* can be paired with the song "The Wheels on the Bus" to teach the spelling and recognition of the word. The melody of the song can be paired with the following lyrics to teach the spelling and recognition of the word *red*; see the example below for an illustration.

- The letters in the word red, *r-e-d, r-e-d, r-e-d,* the letters in the word red, *r-e-d,* that's how we spell red.

Next, create manipulatives for the older adult participants to use during the group. The manipulatives should contain the word in large print along with additional information to assist in learning the words. For example, the word *red* may be spelled in red ink, or the word *up* may include a picture of an arrow pointing up. Finally, if possible, create a gesture that can accompany the word, such as pointing up for the word *up*, or pointing to self for the word *me*.

Activity Direction: Meet with the older adult participants for 10–15 minutes before the group begins to teach them the songs and gestures and to pass out the manipulatives. During the group, introduce the songs to the children by singing the new lyrics to the song, while the music therapist and older adults perform the gesture and point to the individual letters in the word. Next, form small groups with one or two older adult participants and a few children. During this time, have the older adult participants serve as a group leader and rehearse and reinforce the words with the child participants. After the small group time, reassemble all participants for review in the large group setting. Begin to fade the music and ask children to identify the words without the melody. Eventually use flash cards without the additional clues (pictures, color, etc.) to determine the children's recall of the words.

Clinical Application 4.2

Target Behavior–Younger Generation: Improve academic skills (recognition of primary colors)

Target Behavior–Older Generation: Provide an opportunity to serve as a mentor for young children

Music: Choose music from a variety of familiar and simple children's songs that pertain to colors. This type of music is often found in sections of stores and websites that pertain to academic learning skills for children.

Level 1—General Staff

Activity Name: "Learning Colors"

Advanced Preparation: Identify children's songs that include colors in the lyrics. Locate audio recordings for the songs you will use during the intergenerational activity. Some children's songs with colors also have a board book to accompany the song, such as "Brown Bear, Brown Bear, What Do You See?" and "Five Green and Speckled Frogs." If unable to locate or purchase a board book, create your own by finding pictures to match the color items in the lyrics. In addition, create large cutouts of the item of color for older adult participants to hold. For example, for the song "Five Green and Speckled Frogs," create enough green frogs for every older adult participant to hold.

Activity Direction: Introduce the song to the intergenerational group by playing the audio recording of the song while following along with the board book. Announce to the group that they will sing songs about specific colors. Pass out colored cutouts to the older adult participants and explain that they will point to or hold up the cutout whenever that color is sung during the song. Play the audio recording and encourage all participants to sing while the older adult participants point to or hold up the colored cutout.

Level 2—Volunteer Musician

Activity Name: "Scarf Dancing"

Advanced Preparation: Identify and learn a repertoire of children's songs that contain colors in the lyrics. For example, the songs "I Can Sing a Rainbow" or "I Know the Colors in the Rainbow" contain five or more different colors in the lyrics. Collect enough colored scarves for all the child and older adult participants to have a scarf. Be sure to locate colored scarves to match the different colors in the song. If unable to locate scarves, other types of colored materials can be used.

Activity Direction: Hand out colored scarves to the child and older adult participants. Explain to the group that they will sing songs about colors. Direct the child and older adult participants to move their scarves up and down or side to side whenever they hear their color in the song. Lead participants in singing songs while providing an accompaniment on an instrument such as guitar or piano. The older adult participants will serve as models for the children.

Level 3—Board-Certified Music Therapist

Activity Name: "Color Band"

Other Goals Addressed–Younger Generation: Increase Positive Attitude toward Aging, Increase Prosocial Behaviors, Increase Children's Level of Comfort Interacting with Older Adults

Other Goals Addressed–Older Generation: Increase Meaningful Interactions, Increase Feelings of Usefulness, Increase Feelings of Generativity (Generativity is a measure of psychosocial well-being defined by Erik Erikson as a desire in adults to be concerned with or to contribute something to a younger generation.)

Advanced Preparation: Gather enough colored instruments such as egg shakers, maracas, etc. for the intergenerational group. Create an original simple song or a piggyback song version of a familiar children's song such as "The Hokey Pokey" or "If You're Happy and You Know It." The lyrics to the song should contain directions of when or how to play a colored instrument. The example below is an illustration of piggyback lyrics for the song "The Hokey Pokey."

- Shake your green egg up, shake your green egg down, shake your green egg up then shake it all around. You shake your eggs together and you shake them really loud. That's what it's all about.

The example below is an illustration of piggyback lyrics for the song "If You're Happy and You Know It."

- If you have a blue egg, shake it now. If you have a blue egg, shake it now. If you have a blue egg, then shake and shake and shake. If you have a blue egg, shake it now.

Activity Direction: Meet with the older adult participants 10–15 minutes before the intergenerational group and explain the purpose of the upcoming session. Practice the activity with the older adult participants to provide comfort and familiarity with the activity. During the group, hand out colored instruments to the participants. Lead the participants in singing while accompanying the group on guitar or piano. Be sure to use music qualities such as tempo, volume, and chords to emphasize the color. Depending on the size of the group, have one or more older adults responsible for one color. When handing out the instruments, use that time to reinforce and teach color concepts. Next, form small groups with one or two older adults working with a few children. During the small group, allow the older adult participants to review the color concepts learned in the song. After the small group work, return to the large group setting and review the song and color concepts once more. After this final review, begin to fade the music and identify examples in the classroom environment that are the same colors that were learned on that day. For a follow-up question, ask children to think of other colors such as things outdoors, food, things at their home, or colors that they are wearing.

Clinical Application 4.3

Target Behavior–Younger Generation: Improve prosocial behavior

Target Behavior–Older Generation: Decrease isolation

Music: Choose music from genres that are familiar to both generations. Some possible genres are folk songs, patriotic songs, and show tunes. Factors such as ethnicity, culture, and ages of the younger and older generation may affect the genres of music that are familiar to both generations.

Level 1—General Staff

Activity Name: "Song Title Mix Up"

Advanced Preparation: Locate recordings and song titles that are familiar to both generations. Shuffle the words in the song title so that it is unrecognizable. For example, the song "You Are My Sunshine" may read, *My Sunshine Are You*. Create a list of mixed-up song titles. Gather a dry erase board or a large poster board to write on during the activity.

Activity Direction: Divide the group into older adult and child dyads. Start the activity by writing the scrambled song title on the board. Have the older adult and child dyads work together to determine the correct title. Once the title is correctly guessed, play the song selection and encourage participants to sing. Keep score for the dyads to determine an overall winner.

Level 2—Volunteer Musician

Activity Name: "Name That Tune"

Advanced Preparation: Create a few song categories that represent the music selections on your repertoire list. For example, your repertoire may be arranged by the following categories: patriotic songs, songs with a color in it, songs about a state, songs with the letter "I," songs with a boy's name, etc. For this activity, you will need to locate sheet music with the melody line for each song. Next, mark your music in 5-note increments for ease in leading the activity with the group.

Activity Direction: For this activity, divide the intergenerational group into child and older adult dyads. Explain the directions of the game. Once the group is divided into teams, begin the game with two intergenerational dyads. Select one song category for dyads, such as a patriotic song, and allow dyad 1 to say how many notes they need to hear in order for them to name the song. Dyad 2 will then decide that they can name the song in fewer notes or they can tell dyad 1 to name the song. This will continue until one dyad tells the other to "name that tune." Encourage interaction between the younger and older participants. Once a number of notes are identified, play that number of notes from the melody on piano, guitar, or other instrument. Allow each dyad 60 seconds to guess the name of the song. If the dyad identifies the name of the song correctly, they receive 1 point; if the song is not correctly identified, the other team is allowed to guess the name of the song and receive 1 point. If neither team correctly identifies the song title, allow the rest of the participants to guess the song title. Once the correct song title is identified, sing a verse and/or chorus of the song. Keep score for all the participants.

Level 3—Board-Certified Music Therapist

Activity Name: "Song Writing"

Other Goals Addressed–Younger Generation: Increase Positive Attitude toward Aging, Increase Children's Level of Comfort Interacting with Older Adults

Other Goals Addressed–Older Generation: Increase Meaningful Interactions, Increase Feelings of Usefulness, Increase Feelings of Generativity (Generativity is a measure of psychosocial well-being defined by Erik Erikson as a desire in adults to be concerned with or to contribute something to a younger generation.)

Advanced Preparation: For this activity, select a theme that participants will write a song about, such as hobbies, emotions, family, friends, etc. You may select a song with the specific theme or compose a song of your own. Songs that are repetitive or have a simple musical form such as blues or ABA form are helpful for songwriting. In addition, develop a question that relates to the theme of the song for intergenerational participants to discuss. Answers to the question will form the lyrics for the songwriting activity. An example of a repetitive song that works well for songwriting is "I Love the Mountains." One question that relates to the lyrics of the song is to ask participants to discuss their hobbies.

Activity Direction: Teach the song to the participants. Once the group has learned the song, divide them into intergenerational dyads. Direct participants to answer the theme question during the dyad interactions. After the dyad discussion, lead the group in a fill-in-the-blank songwriting activity with their responses from the theme question. Depending on the size of the group, this can be done as one large group or several small groups consisting of two to three intergenerational dyads. These smaller groups can take turns singing their verse for the entire group. If time is an issue, each dyad can be responsible for one line of the song.

Clinical Application 4.4

Target Behavior–Younger Generation: Improve prosocial behavior

Target Behavior–Older Generation: Decrease isolation

Music: Choose rhythmic and fast tempo music that may be familiar to both generations. Some possible genres are folk songs, patriotic songs, and show tunes. Factors such as ethnicity, culture, and ages of the younger and older generation may affect the genres of music that are familiar to both generations.

Level 1—General Staff

Activity Name: "Intergenerational Band"

Advanced Preparation: Gather two or more different types of musical instruments. Egg shakers work well in addition to rhythm sticks, drums, or maracas. If you do not have access to instruments, be creative, and use other materials such as bowls, pots, lids, etc. Be sure to think about safety when selecting possible instruments for both the children and older adults. Collect recordings of various songs and bring them to the intergenerational group.

Activity Direction: To begin the activity, pass out the instruments or let the participants choose their own. Lead the intergenerational band in playing along with recorded music. After one or two songs, have the participants switch instruments with one another. Continue until all of the participants have played at least two different instruments during the group.

Level 2—Volunteer Musician

Activity Name: "Intergenerational Band"

Advanced Preparation: Gather rhythm or kitchen band instruments (see Level 1 for ideas). Choose songs that have a chorus and verse pattern or songs that are highly repetitive. Learn songs on an accompaniment instrument or bring recordings of the songs to the intergenerational session.

Activity Direction: To begin, sing the song through once using one verse and one chorus. Next, divide participants into two groups, one group that plays on the chorus and one group that plays on the verse. Sing the song through again with each group playing at the correct place. If time permits, allow the participants to switch instruments and to alternate playing on the verse or chorus.

Level 3—Board-Certified Music Therapist

Activity Name: "Drum Circle"

Other Goals Addressed–Younger Generation: Improve Positive Attitude toward Aging, Increase Children's Level of Comfort Interacting with Older Adults

Other Goals Addressed–Older Generation: Increase Meaningful Interactions, Increase Feelings of Usefulness, Increase Feelings of Generativity (Generativity is a measure of psychosocial well-being defined by Erik Erikson as a desire in adults to be concerned with or to contribute something to a younger generation.)

Advanced Preparation: Identify a recorded song that has a steady rhythmic pattern. Create two rhythm patterns that will fit the song. Gather drums and mallets for all of the participants.

Activity Direction: Divide the group into child and older adult dyads. Pass out one drum and one mallet to each dyad. Identify one generation as the instrument holder and the other generation as the instrument player. Teach the entire group rhythm 1, allowing both generations to have a turn as instrument holder and player. Repeat this process to teach the entire group rhythm 2. Once participants can successfully play each rhythm, introduce the recorded song and alternate between playing rhythm 1 and rhythm 2 and between instrument holder and player. If the group is progressing, divide the group in two and have one group play rhythm 1 and the other group play rhythm 2. Once they are successful without music, add the recorded music.

FOCUS AREA 2: EMPLOYING MUSIC IN A YOUNGER GENERATION SERVING OLDER GENERATION MODEL

Clinical Application 4.5

Target Behavior–Younger Generation: Improve willingness to interact with older adults

Target Behavior–Older Generation: Improve attitude toward younger generation

Music: Choose music from an electronic game that will be familiar to younger and older participants. Depending on the age of the participants, music may be selected from classical, popular, big band genres, and more. Factors such as ethnicity, culture, and ages of the younger and older generation may affect the genres of music that are familiar to both generations.

Level 1—General Staff

Activity Name: "Rhythm Games"

Advanced Preparation: Purchase the game Donkey Konga. Donkey Konga is a music-based game that uses instruments (two bongo drums) to move a character. Music used in the game includes classical songs and big band tunes that may be familiar to the older adult participants.

Activity Direction: Meet with the younger participants to teach game objectives. Assign each younger participant to an older adult participant to form intergenerational dyads. Have the younger participants teach the older adult participants how to play the game. Once the older adult participants are comfortable playing the game, have the intergenerational dyads compete against one another.

Level 2—Volunteer Musician

Activity Name: "Rhythm Games"

Advanced Preparation: Purchase the game Donkey Konga. Donkey Konga is a music-based game that uses instruments (two bongo drums) to move a character. Music includes classical songs and big band tunes that may be familiar to the older adult participants. Locate audio recordings of the songs used in the game.

Activity Direction: Meet with the younger participants to teach game objectives. Assign each younger participant to an older adult participant to form intergenerational dyads. Have the younger participants teach the older adult participants how to play the game. Once the older adult participants are comfortable playing the game, have the intergenerational dyads compete against one another. Next, lead the intergenerational group in a listening activity. Play the original audio recordings of the songs used in the game and lead the group in a discussion on the differences in the video game recordings and the audio recordings you brought to the activity.

Level 3—Board-Certified Music Therapist

Activity Name: "Adapted Music Lessons"

Other Goals Addressed–Younger Generation: Improve Prosocial Behaviors, Increase Positive Attitude toward Aging

Other Goals Addressed–Older Generation: Decrease Isolation, Increase Meaningful Interactions, Increase Connection to Society through Learning Technology

Advanced Preparation: Contact a music instructor at a nearby school, such as a high school or college, to determine if there are any students interested in a community service project. The community service project will last a semester during which the students will teach older adults adapted music lessons. Have the music instructor identify the number of students and the type of instruments that will be available for lessons. At the same time, identify and recruit older adults who are interested in learning how to play a new musical instrument. Work with the music teacher to locate music stores to rent instruments that will be used for the program. Create a syllabus with the music instructor and students pertaining to the adapted music lessons. The final project will be a concert with the younger and older participants. The music therapist and the teacher should work together to determine repertoire that older adults will be successful in learning during the program. Teach students about sensory changes that occur with aging and other areas of concern that students may need to be sensitive to, such as cultural differences, age range, and physical or cognitive changes.

Activity Direction: During this project you will serve as the coordinator between the music teacher, students, and older adults, as well as a role model for the students on appropriate teaching styles when working with an older adult population. Once your schedule is in place, be sure to remind older adults of their lesson time. Also, during the week you can check in with the older adults regarding their practice schedule and progress. During lesson times, rotate through the different sessions to observe the intergenerational lessons. After the weekly lesson, you should allow at least 15 minutes to speak with students about their progress and any concerns. The final outcome for this project will be a performance.

Clinical Application 4.6

Target Behavior–Younger Generation: Improve willingness to interact with older adults

Target Behavior–Older Generation: Improve attitude toward younger generation

Music: Select music based on the preferred music of the older participants. Depending on the age of the participants, music may be selected from classical, oldies, big band genres, and more. Factors such as ethnicity, culture, and ages of the older generation may affect the genres of music that are familiar.

Level 1—General Staff

Activity Name: "Music Technology/Computer Buddies"

Advanced Preparation: Create a sign-up sheet for the older adult participants to learn how to use iTunes, YouTube, Pandora, and other music listening/purchasing applications on the Internet. Contact the leader of the organization where you will obtain younger participant volunteers. Discuss ways that the younger participants can teach older adult participants how to use the different websites. Assist the younger participants in creating a lesson plan for their teaching program. Obtain all the materials that younger participants will need. Ask each older participant to identify a favorite song.

Activity Direction: As the participants arrive, have each older adult participant write down a favorite song. Introduce the younger and older participants to each other. Let the younger participants lead the demonstration on how to use the music applications. Allow time for the older participants to share their favorite song and for the younger participants to find the song using the Internet application.

Level 2—Volunteer Musician

Activity Name: "Music Technology/Computer Buddies"

Advanced Preparation: Create a sign-up sheet for older adult participants to learn how to use iTunes, YouTube, Pandora, and other music listening/purchasing applications on the Internet. Contact the leader of the organization where you will obtain younger participant volunteers. Discuss ways that the younger participants can teach older adult participants how to use the different websites. Assist younger participants in creating a lesson plan for their teaching program. Obtain all materials that younger participants will need. Ask each older participant to identify a favorite song.

Activity Direction: As the participants arrive, have each older adult participant write down a favorite song. Introduce younger and older participants to each other. Let the younger participants lead the demonstration on how to use the music applications. Allow time for older participants to share their favorite song, and for the younger participants to find the song using the Internet application.

Level 3—Board-Certified Music Therapist

Activity Name: "Music Technology/Computer Buddies"

Other Goals Addressed–Younger Generation: Improve Prosocial Behaviors, Increase Positive Attitude toward Aging

Other Goals Addressed–Older Generation: Decrease Isolation, Increase Meaningful Interactions, Increase Connection to Society through Learning Technology

Advanced Preparation: Create a sign-up sheet for older adult participants to learn how to use iTunes, YouTube, Pandora, and other music listening/purchasing applications on the Internet. Contact the leader of the organization where you will obtain younger participant volunteers.

Discuss ways that the younger participants can teach older adult participants how to use the different websites. Determine how many sessions the group will meet. Lead a discussion group regarding sensitivity to aging issues, preferred music of older adults, and other specifics about the older adult participants, such as sensory changes and assistive devices. Assist younger participants in creating a lesson plan for their teaching program. Obtain all materials that younger participants will need. Ask each older participant to identify a favorite song. Create questions for the younger participants to ask the older participants to assist with a structured conversation intervention. Questions can pertain to older adults' music preferences, hobbies, prior professions, etc.

Activity Direction: As the participants arrive, have each older adult participant write down a favorite song. Introduce younger and older participants to each other. Let the younger participants lead the demonstration on how to use the music applications. Allow time for older participants to share their favorite song, and for the younger participants to find the song using the Internet application. After locating the song, provide the younger participants with questions to foster interaction during the structured conversation intervention.

Clinical Application 4.7

Target Behavior–Younger Generation: Improve willingness to interact with older adults

Target Behavior–Older Generation: Improve attitude toward younger generation

Music: Select music that is upbeat and rhythmic to accompany the line dances.

Level 1—General Staff

Activity Name: "Music Dancing"

Advanced Preparation: Locate an organization providing services to young people that is interested in participating in an intergenerational program. Contact the leader of the organization where you will obtain younger participant volunteers. Explain to the leader of the organization that the younger participants will teach a simple line dance to older adult participants. Work with the leader to determine an appropriate line dance for the older adult participants, noting that adaptations may need to be made depending on participants' level of physical functioning. Obtain music needed for the line dance.

Activity Direction: First, let the younger participants demonstrate the line dance for the older adult participants with music. Next, direct the younger participants to teach the older participants the individual steps to the dance. Once the dance is learned, pair it with music.

Level 2—Volunteer Musician

Activity Name: "Music Dancing"

Advanced Preparation: Locate an organization providing services to young people that is interested in participating in an intergenerational program. Contact the leader of the organization where you will obtain younger participant volunteers. Work with the leader to determine an appropriate line dance for the older adult participants, noting that adaptations may need to be made depending on the participants' level of physical functioning. Obtain music needed for the line dance.

Activity Direction: First, let the younger participants demonstrate the line dance for the older adult participants with music. Next, direct the younger participants to teach the older participants individual steps to the dance. Once the dance is learned, pair it with music. If possible, provide live accompaniment of music to the dance. Serve as a model and provide assistance where needed.

Level 3—Board-Certified Music Therapist

Activity Name: "Music Dancing"

Other Goals Addressed–Younger Generation: Improve Prosocial Behaviors, Increase Positive Attitude toward Aging

Other Goals Addressed–Older Generation: Decrease Isolation, Increase Meaningful Interactions, Increase Connection to Society

Advanced Preparation: Locate an organization providing services to young people that is interested in participating in an intergenerational program. Contact the leader of the organization where you will obtain younger participant volunteers. Work with the leader to determine an appropriate line dance for the older adult participants, noting that adaptations may need to be made depending on participants' level of physical functioning. Obtain music needed for the line dance. Have the younger generation prepare two dances: a dance that is familiar to the younger generation, and a dance that is familiar to the older generation.

Activity Direction: First, let the younger participants demonstrate the line dance for the older adult participants with music. Next, direct the younger participants to teach the older participants individual steps to the dance. Once the dance is learned, pair it with music. If possible, provide live accompaniment of music to the dance. Serve as a model and provide assistance where needed. Direct the younger participants to teach the second dance using the steps described above. End with leading the group in a reminiscence intervention pertaining to dances from the older generations' younger years, including dances from special occasions like weddings, parties, and more. Compare favorite and popular dances of the younger participants to favorite and popular dances of the older participants.

Clinical Application 4.8

Target Behavior–Younger Generation: Improve willingness to interact with older adults

Target Behavior–Older Generation: Improve attitude toward younger generation

Music: Ask the music director of a music group comprised of young people to select a few songs that are familiar to the older adults in your setting. Depending on the age of the participants, music may be selected from classical, oldies, big band genres, and more. Factors such as ethnicity, culture, and ages of the older generation may affect the genres of music that are familiar.

Level 1—General Staff

Activity Name: "Music Performance"

Advanced Preparation: Contact the director of a music group comprised of young people to perform at your facility. Ask the director to include a song that is familiar to the older adult participants. Identify any needs that the performing group will have. Advertise the upcoming program at the facility.

Activity Direction: Introduce the younger participants to the older participants. Encourage the older participants to sing or hum along to songs that are familiar. After the performance, encourage the younger and older participants to interact with each other.

Level 2—Volunteer Musician

Activity Name: "Music Performance"

Advanced Preparation: Contact the director of a music group comprised of young people to perform at your facility. Ask the director to include a song that you accompany that is familiar to the older adult participants. Song suggestions can include songs with a specific theme such as summertime or a holiday. Identify any needs that the group will have. Advertise the upcoming program at the facility.

Activity Direction: Introduce the younger participants to the older participants. Accompany the music group on the selected familiar song. Encourage the older participants to sing or hum along to the song that is familiar to them. After the performance, encourage the younger and older participants to interact with each other.

Level 3—Board-Certified Music Therapist

Activity Name: "Singing Telegram"

Other Goals Addressed–Younger Generation: Improve Prosocial Behaviors, Increase Positive Attitude toward Aging

Other Goals Addressed–Older Generation: Decrease Isolation, Increase Positive Interaction within Environment

Advanced Preparation: Contact the director of a music group comprised of young people to perform at your facility during a holiday such as Valentine's Day. Work with the director and the music group to teach a few older adult love songs that are familiar to the older adults at your facility. Choose songs that are short, familiar, and easy to learn, such as "I Love You Truly" or "Let Me Call You Sweetheart." Advertise the singing telegram program and encourage older adults to send singing telegrams to other residents and staff at the facility. Create a sign-up form that includes the sender's name, recipient's name, and room number. Choose a specific time for the singing telegrams to occur, for example, 10:00–11:00 a.m.

Activity Direction: On the day of the singing telegrams, meet with the younger participants to rehearse the love songs. Lead the younger singers around the building to deliver singing telegrams. This activity can be adapted for other holidays such as Thanksgiving, Christmas, 4th of July, etc.

FOCUS AREA 3: EMPLOYING MUSIC IN AN OLDER GENERATION AND YOUNGER GENERATION LEARNING-TOGETHER MODEL

Clinical Application 4.9

Target Behavior–Younger Generation: Improve acceptance of older adults

Target Behavior–Older Generation: Improve quality of life

Music: For this activity you may select songs that are either unfamiliar or familiar to the younger or older generation. Factors such as ethnicity, culture, and ages of the younger and older generation may affect the genres of music that are familiar to both generations.

Level 1—General Staff

Activity Name: "Cover Songs vs. Original Songs"

Advanced Preparation: Many original songs have been remade into cover songs by different artists. Often times, the cover song will be recorded by an artist in a different genre. For example, the song "I Will Always Love You" was originally sung by Dolly Parton as a country song, yet the same song became popular again when Whitney Houston recorded a pop ballad rendition. For this activity, locate recordings of songs performed by two different artists. Preferably, find songs that are recorded by different artists performed in different genres. Another example of a cover song is "I Can't Help Falling in Love with You," a song performed by Elvis Presley and UB40. Try to find songs that are different, such as slow versus fast, or a solo voice versus a group performance. Find any trivia related to the songs, such as the date, information about the performers, and more.

Activity Direction: Select a song and play both versions of the recordings for the participants. Next, ask the group to identify which audio version is familiar to them. During this activity, also ask the participants to vote on which version of the song they prefer and discuss reasons for their preferences. Share any trivia found with the group regarding the songs and artists/performers.

Level 2—Volunteer Musician

Activity Name: "Cover Songs vs. Original Songs"

Advanced Preparation: Many original songs have been remade into cover songs by different artists. Often times the cover song will be recorded by an artist in a different genre. For example, the song "I Will Always Love You" was originally sung by Dolly Parton as a country song, yet the same song became popular again when Whitney Houston recorded a pop ballad rendition. For this activity, locate recordings of songs performed by two different artists. Preferably, find songs that are recorded by different artists performed in different genres. Another example of a cover song is "I Can't Help Falling in Love with You," a song performed by Elvis Presley and UB40. Try to find songs that are different, such as slow versus fast, or a solo voice versus a group performance. Find any trivia related to the songs, such as the date, information about the performers, and more. Learn both versions of the songs on an accompaniment instrument. Prepare lyric sheets of the songs for the participants.

Activity Direction: Select a song and play both versions of the recordings for the participants. Next, ask the group to identify which audio version is familiar to them. Also ask the participants to vote on which version of the song they prefer and discuss their choices. Share any trivia found with the group regarding the songs and artists/performers. Lead the participants in singing a verse and/or chorus of each version of the song while playing an accompaniment instrument.

Level 3—Board-Certified Music Therapist

Activity Name: "Music History"

Other Goals Addressed–Younger Generation: Improve Willingness to Interact with Older Adults, Improve Positive Attitude toward Aging

Other Goals Addressed–Older Generation: Decrease Isolation, Improve Life Satisfaction, Increase Opportunities for Social Interaction

Advanced Preparation: Interview the younger and older participants to identify their favorite artists, music styles, and songs. Create a music history lesson based on the preferred music interview. Include visual and audio examples of the music. Determine the number of sessions for the music history class and divide information among sessions. Locate audio recordings of the songs and videos that are popular and representative of the genre you are teaching.

Activity Direction: Allow each participant to introduce his or her favorite song, artist, and/or music style. Play audio selection and have participants share why that song means something to them. Follow the music listening with a brief music history lesson about the music style and artists. Include audio and video examples of other songs that fit the artist and style.

Clinical Application 4.10

Target Behavior–Younger Generation: Improve acceptance of older adults

Target Behavior–Older Generation: Improve quality of life

Music: Identify songs that will be familiar to both generations. You can select songs that are from different genres and have various tempos. Depending on the age of the participants, music may be selected from classical, popular, children's tunes, big band genres, and more. Factors such as ethnicity, culture, and ages of the younger and older generation may affect the genres of music that are familiar to both generations.

Level 1—General Staff

Activity Name: "Karaoke Singing"

Advanced Preparation: Purchase karaoke equipment if it is not available at your facility. Select karaoke CDs from various decades that will be familiar to the younger and older generations. For older adult participants, select music from 1900–1950s based on music preferences of the groups. For the younger participants, select music from their preferred style and decade. Create a list of songs available for participants to choose from during the karaoke activity. You may want to create a master list of songs with the CD and track number for ease of locating the songs during the activity. Also create song slips for participants to write down their name and song selection.

Activity Direction: Pass out song lists to the participants. Allow time for each participant to select a song to sing and fill out the song slip. Collect all song slips and place in a container. Randomly select one song slip at a time to choose a participant. You can also encourage partner and group performances for those who may be hesitant to sing alone.

Level 2—Volunteer Musician

Activity Name: "Karaoke Singing"

Advanced Preparation: Purchase karaoke equipment if it is not available at the facility. Select karaoke CDs from various decades that will be familiar to younger and older generations. For older participants, select music from 1900–1950s based on music preferences of the groups. For the younger participants, select music from their preferred style and decade. Create a list of songs available for participants to choose from. You may want to create a master list of songs with the CD and track number for ease of locating songs during the activity. Also create song slips for participants to write down their name and song selection.

Activity Direction: Pass out song lists to participants. Allow time for each participant to select a song to sing and fill out song slip. Collect all song slips and place in a container. Randomly select a song slip to choose a participant. You can also encourage partner and group performances for those who may be hesitant to sing alone.

Level 3—Board-Certified Music Therapist

Activity Name: "Intergenerational Choir"

Other Goals Addressed–Younger Generation: Improve Willingness to Interact with Older Adults, Improve Positive Attitude toward Aging

Other Goals Addressed–Older Generation: Decrease Isolation, Improve Life Satisfaction, Increase Opportunities for Social Interaction

Advanced Preparation: Determine the genres and music selections that the intergenerational choir will sing. Some choirs have used music that is familiar to both generations, such as Broadway songs, music of the younger and older generations, popular/contemporary music from each generation, resulting in each generation learning a few new songs. Some choirs have also used one genre, such as rock music, to direct the group. Recruit older and younger participants to join the intergenerational choir. Locate music, audio recordings, and lyrics for the songs. Create song sheets or print words on a large flip chart. Determine what accompaniment instrument you will use for each song. Also, plan and implement alternate music activities that will foster interaction between the younger and older generations.

Activity Direction: Arrange the chairs in rows or arcs. Plan for seating arrangements to include younger participants intermixed with older participants to foster cross-age interactions. Pass out the lyrics to all choir members. Teach the songs using a variety of methods such as music listening, chaining, and repetition. Have the choir perform a number of musical selections for a final concert.

Clinical Application 4.11

Target Behavior–Younger Generation: Improve acceptance of older adults

Target Behavior–Older Generation: Improve quality of life

Music: The book *Group Rhythm and Drumming with Older Adults: Music Therapy Techniques and Multimedia Training Guide* and accompanying DVD provide information on music and instruments needed for each activity. Therefore, music and materials will be determined based on the activity used in the group.

Level 1—General Staff

Activity Name: "Group Drumming"

Advanced Preparation: Purchase the book *Group Rhythm and Drumming with Older Adults: Music Therapy Techniques and Multimedia Training Guide* by Barbara Reuer, Barbara Crowe, and Barry Bernstein (available from the AMTA). This book and DVD contain a training section, warm-up activities that can be performed with the DVD, and drumming activities that are not accompanied by the DVD. Determine which activities you would like to use, what materials you may need, and the DVD sections to use. Each activity is described in the book as well as on the DVD. Practice the activity so that you can model and/or lead the participants.

Activity Direction: Pass out instruments to the participants. Briefly explain the object of the music activity. Turn on the DVD clip for the warm-up activity. Model the various instrument playing techniques from the DVD for the participants. When comfortable, lead the participants through the drumming/rhythm activities that do not use the DVD.

Level 2—Volunteer Musician

Activity Name: "Group Drumming"

Advanced Preparation: Purchase the book *Group Rhythm and Drumming with Older Adults: Music Therapy Techniques and Multimedia Training Guide* by Barbara Reuer, Barbara Crowe, and Barry Bernstein (available from the AMTA). This book and DVD contain a training section, warm-up activities that can be performed with the DVD, and drumming activities that are not accompanied by the DVD. Determine which activities you would like to use, what materials you may need, and the DVD sections to use. Each activity is described in the book as well as on the DVD. Practice the activity so that you can model and/or lead the participants.

Activity Direction: Pass out instruments to the participants. Briefly explain the object of the music activity. Turn on the DVD clip for the warm-up activity. Model the various instrument playing techniques from the DVD for the participants. When comfortable, lead the participants through the drumming/rhythm activities that do not use the DVD.

Level 3—Board-Certified Music Therapist

Activity Name: "Tone Chime Ensemble"

Other Goals Addressed–Younger Generation: Improve Willingness to Interact with Older Adults, Improve Positive Attitude toward Aging

Other Goals Addressed–Older Generation: Decrease Isolation, Improve Life Satisfaction, Increase Opportunities for Social Interaction

Advanced Preparation: This intervention allows participants to play either the melody of a song or an accompaniment pattern based on chords or an ostinato pattern. Depending on the size of the group and the number of octaves contained in your tone chime set, it may be easier to play chords or an ostinato pattern (for a larger group) or the melody (for a smaller group). Once songs are selected, create large-print lyric sheets that contain symbols to indicate when participants should play (i.e., chord qualities—I or IV, group names—group 1 or group 2, or colors—red group or green group). For example, you may want to use a three-chord song that uses a I, IV, and V chord. You can divide the large group into three sections/small groups and assign each smaller group to a chord; group 1 can play the I chord, group 2 can play the IV chord, and group 3 can play the V chord.

Activity Direction: Teach the participants how to play the tone chimes, checking for a clear ringing sound. Once everyone is comfortable playing the instruments, teach participants either the chorus or verse of the song. Utilize chaining, repetition, and other teaching elements for participants to learn the music.

Clinical Application 4.12

Target Behavior–Younger Generation: Improve acceptance of older adults

Target Behavior–Older Generation: Improve quality of life

Music: Select songs that are familiar to both generations. Depending on the age of the participants, music may be selected from classical, oldies, popular, children's tunes, big band genres, and more. Factors such as ethnicity, culture, and ages of the younger and older generation may affect the genres of music that are familiar to both generations.

Level 1—General Staff

Activity Name: "Instrument Making"

Advanced Preparation: Search the Internet for instructions on how to make rhythm instruments. Some instruments that are easy to make are egg shakers, tambourines, rain sticks, and drums. Obtain the materials needed for each participant to make a rhythm instrument. Determine how you will set up the room, making sure to plan for enough work surfaces for all participants. Make one instrument ahead of time to serve as a model.

Activity Direction: Divide the participants into younger and older dyads so that both generations have the opportunity to work together. Show participants the instrument that they will create during the activity. Demonstrate and provide step-by-step instructions to the participants on how to create the instrument with the materials provided. Provide assistance as needed to group members. When the instruments are completed, provide an opportunity for each participant to play his or her instrument.

Level 2—Volunteer Musician

Activity Name: "Instrument Making"

Advanced Preparation: Search the Internet for instructions on how to make rhythm instruments. Some instruments that are easy to make are egg shakers, tambourines, rain sticks, and drums. Obtain the materials needed for each participant to make a rhythm instrument. Determine how you will set up the room, making sure to plan for enough work surfaces for all participants. Make one instrument ahead of time to serve as a model. Select a song for participants to sing and accompany with their newly created instruments.

Activity Direction: Divide the participants into younger and older dyads so that both generations have the opportunity to work together. Show participants the instrument that they will create during the activity. Demonstrate and provide step-by-step instructions to the participants on how to create the instrument with the materials provided. Provide assistance to the group as needed. When instruments are completed, provide an opportunity for each participant to play his or her instrument. Additionally, lead the group in using their newly created instruments to accompany and sing a familiar song.

Level 3—Board-Certified Music Therapist

Activity Name: "Instrument Making"

Other Goals Addressed–Younger Generation: Improve Willingness to Interact with Older Adults, Improve Positive Attitude toward Aging

Other Goals Addressed–Older Generation: Decrease Isolation, Improve Life Satisfaction, Increase Opportunities for Social Interaction

Advanced Preparation: Search the Internet for instructions on how to make rhythm instruments. Some instruments that are easy to make are egg shakers, tambourines, rain sticks, and drums. Obtain the materials needed for each participant to make a rhythm instrument. Determine how you will set up the room, making sure to plan for enough work surfaces for all participants. Make one instrument ahead of time to serve as a model. Create rhythmic accompaniment patterns for a drum circle.

Activity Direction: Divide participants into younger and older dyads so that both generations have the opportunity to work together. Show participants the instrument that they will be creating. Allow each pair to create two instruments together. Demonstrate and provide step-by-step instructions to participants on how to create the instrument with the materials provided. Provide assistance to the group as needed. When instruments are completed, provide an opportunity for each participant to play his or her instrument. Next, lead participants in a drum circle, utilizing call and response, repetition, and chaining techniques to teach various rhythms. Follow activities with a discussion of teamwork and the process of making instruments together.

FOCUS AREA 4: EMPLOYING MUSIC IN AN OLDER GENERATION AND YOUNGER GENERATION RECREATIONAL MODEL

Clinical Application 4.13

Target Behavior–Younger Generation: Increase frequency of positive interactions with older adults

Target Behavior–Older Generation: Increase frequency of positive interactions with younger persons

Music: Choose music from an electronic game that will be familiar to younger and older participants. Depending on the age of the participants, music may be selected from classical, popular, children's tunes, big band genres, and more. Factors such as ethnicity, culture, and ages of the younger and older generation may affect the genres of music that are familiar to both generations.

Level 1—General Staff

Activity Name: "Music Game–Wii Music"

Advanced Preparation: Purchase the Wii Music system to use with the intergenerational group. Look through the directions and various applications of the system. Wii Music contains 50 songs and over 60 instruments. Choose songs that are familiar to both generations, such as classical and folk songs. Determine how many instruments to use for the activity based on how many older and younger participants will be in the group. For a small group, each older and younger participant can play a different instrument and part. For a larger group, pair older and younger participants together for each instrument or part.

Activity Direction: Set-up the Wii Music system and chairs in an arrangement that allows all participants to view what is occurring. For a small group, an arc of chairs with the Wii Music system in the middle may be most conducive. For a large group, start with a small arc of chairs for those who will participate at one time. Then add an additional row of chairs for the rest of the participants behind the small arc. Use the on-screen gaming directions to teach the participants how to use the game controllers to create sounds. Model movements for the participants and assist anyone who is having difficulty. Follow the on-screen directions to play familiar songs selected for the group. Provide assistance and encouragement to the younger and older participants as needed.

Level 2—Volunteer Musician

Activity Name: "Music Game–Wii Music"

Advanced Preparation: Purchase the Wii Music system to use with the intergenerational group. Look through the directions and various applications. Wii Music contains 50 songs and over 60 instruments. Choose songs that are familiar to both generations, such as classical and folk songs. Determine how many instruments to use for the activity based on how many older and younger participants will be in the group. For a small group, each older and younger participant can play a different instrument and part. For a larger group, pair older and younger participants together for each instrument or part.

Activity Direction: Set-up the Wii Music system and chairs in an arrangement that allows all participants to view what is occurring. For a small group, an arc of chairs with the Wii Music system in the middle may be most conducive. For a large group, start with a small arc of chairs for those who will participate at one time. Then add an additional row of chairs for the rest of the participants behind the small arc. Use the on-screen gaming directions to teach participants how to use the game controllers to create sounds. Model movements for the participants and assist anyone who is having difficulty. Follow the on-screen directions to play familiar songs selected for the group. Provide assistance and encouragement to the younger and older participants as needed.

Level 3—Board-Certified Music Therapist

Activity Name: "Music Game–Wii Music"

Other Goals Addressed–Younger Generation: Improve Social Acceptance of Older Adults, Improve Attitudes toward Older Adults

Other Goals Addressed–Older Generation: Decrease Isolation, Improve Meaningful Interactions, Improve Attitudes toward Younger Persons

Advanced Preparation: Purchase the Wii Music system to use with the intergenerational group. Look through the directions and various applications. Wii Music contains 50 songs and over 60 instruments. Choose songs that are familiar and unfamiliar to both generations. Create lyric sheets for the selected songs and be prepared to play the songs on an accompaniment instrument. Interview the younger and older participants about their music skill, identifying if they currently play or have played an instrument in the past, as well as what instrument they want to learn how to play. Determine how many instruments to use for the activity based on the responses of the participants. For a small group, each older and younger participant can play a different instrument and part. For a larger group, pair older and younger participants together for each instrument or part.

Activity Direction: Set-up the Wii Music system and chairs in an arrangement that allows all participants to view what is occurring. For a small group, an arc of chairs with the Wii Music system in the middle may be most conducive. For a large group, start with a small arc of chairs for those who will participate at one time. Then add an additional row of chairs for the rest of the participants behind the small arc. Hand out lyric sheets to the participants for songs that will be used with the Wii Music system. Rehearse familiar songs with the group. Also teach unfamiliar songs to the group using chaining techniques. Use the on-screen gaming directions to teach the participants how to use the game controllers to create sounds. Model movements for the participants and assist anyone who is having difficulty. Follow the on-screen directions to play familiar songs selected for the group. Provide assistance and encouragement to the younger and older participants as needed. Lead the group in a discussion that compares and contrasts the Wii instruments to real instruments. Include topics such as sound quality, ease of instrument playing, and more.

Clinical Application 4.14

Target Behavior–Younger Generation: Increase frequency of positive interactions with older adults

Target Behavior–Older Generation: Increase frequency of positive interactions with younger persons

Music: Select songs that are familiar to both generations. Depending on the age of the participants, music may be selected from classical, popular, children's tunes, big band genres, and more. Factors such as ethnicity, culture, and ages of the younger and older generation may affect the genres of music that are familiar to both generations.

Level 1—General Staff

Activity Name: "Music Pictionary"

Advanced Preparation: Identify songs that are familiar to both generations, such as folk and patriotic. If the younger generation contains high school or college students, you can choose popular songs from the 1950s, such as songs by Elvis Presley. Create game cards by typing various song titles on index-card size slips of paper. Song titles should be typed in at least 14-point font. Obtain a dry erase board, eraser, and colored dry erase markers for this activity.

Activity Direction: Divide the intergenerational group into two or more teams. All teams should consist of younger and older participants. Explain the directions of the game to the participants. Let one member of a team (team A) select a game card with a song title printed on it. Next, direct the team member to draw the song title and allow the team 5 minutes to guess the title of the song. If team A correctly identifies the song title, they gain 5 points. If the team is unable to guess the song title or provides an incorrect answer, the other team (team B) has a chance to guess. The other team (team B) will have 1 minute to discuss among themselves the song title. At the end of 1 minute, team B will give one answer. If team B correctly guesses the song title, they receive 2 points. Continue moving among the teams for the remaining time and song titles. At the end of the game, the team with the greatest amount of points is the winner.

Level 2—Volunteer Musician

Activity Name: "Music Pictionary"

Advanced Preparation: Identify songs that are familiar to both generations, such as folk and patriotic. If the younger generation contains high school or college students, you can choose popular songs from the 1950s, such as songs by Elvis Presley. Choose songs that you are comfortable playing on an accompaniment instrument. Create game cards by typing various song titles on index-card size slips of paper. Song titles should be typed in at least 14-point font. Obtain a dry erase board, eraser, and colored dry erase markers for this activity. Also create lyric sheets for the songs used in the activity.

Activity Direction: Divide the intergenerational group into two or more teams. All teams should consist of younger and older participants. Explain the directions of the game to the participants. Let one member of a team (team A) select a game card with a song title printed on it. Next, direct the team member to draw the song title and allow the team 5 minutes to guess the title of the song. If team A correctly identifies the song title, they gain 5 points. If the team is unable to guess the song title or provides an incorrect answer, the other team (team B) has a chance to guess. The other team (team B) will have 1 minute to discuss among themselves the song title. At the end of 1 minute, team B will give one answer. If team B correctly guesses the song title, they receive 2 points. After the song title is guessed, use the song lyrics and an accompaniment instrument to lead participants in singing the song. Continue moving among the teams for the remaining time and song titles. At the end of the game, the team with the greatest amount of points is the winner.

Level 3—Board-Certified Music Therapist

Activity Name: "Music Pictionary"

Other Goals Addressed–Younger Generation: Improve Social Acceptance of Older Adults, Improve Attitudes toward Older Adults

Other Goals Addressed–Older Generation: Decrease Isolation, Improve Meaningful Interactions, Improve Attitudes toward Younger Persons

Advanced Preparation: Identify songs that are familiar to both generations, such as folk and patriotic. If the younger generation contains high school or college students, you can choose popular songs from the 1950s, such as songs by Elvis Presley. Choose songs that you are comfortable playing on an accompaniment instrument. Create game cards by typing various song titles on index-card size slips of paper. Song titles should be typed in at least 14-point font. Obtain a dry erase board, eraser, and colored dry erase markers for this activity. Also create lyric sheets for the songs used in the activity. Identify songs that contain themes for which you can easily create reminiscing questions for the intergenerational participants.

Activity Direction: Divide the intergenerational group into two or more teams. All teams should consist of younger and older participants. Explain the directions of the game to the participants. Let one member of a team (team A) select a game card with a song title printed on it. Next, direct the team member to draw the song title and allow the team 5 minutes to guess the title of the song. If team A correctly identifies the song title, they gain 5 points. If the team is unable to guess the song title or provides an incorrect answer, the other team (team B) has a chance to guess. The other team (team B) will have 1 minute to discuss among themselves the song title. At the end of 1 minute, team B will give one answer. If team B correctly guesses the song title, they receive 2 points. After the song title is guessed, use the song lyrics and an accompaniment instrument to lead participants in singing the song. Use the theme and lyrics of the song to lead the group in reminiscing and discussion. For example, after singing the song "You are My Sunshine," the group can identify things that make them happy. Continue moving among the teams for the remaining time and song titles. At the end of the game, the team with the greatest amount of points is the winner.

Clinical Application 4.15

Target Behavior–Younger Generation: Increase frequency of positive interactions with older adults

Target Behavior–Older Generation: Increase frequency of positive interactions with younger persons

Music: Select music that is familiar to both generations. Depending on the age of the participants, music may be selected from classical, popular, oldies, big band genres, and more. Factors such as ethnicity, culture, and ages of the younger and older generation may affect the genres of music that are familiar to both generations.

Level 1—General Staff

Activity Name: "Musical Charades"

Advanced Preparation: Select a group of songs that are familiar to both generations, such as Broadway musicals, folk, or patriotic music. Choose song titles that are easy to act out in charades. Create game cards on index-card size sheets of paper with the song title printed on it. Locate recordings of the songs.

Activity Direction: Explain the game directions to the group. Include charade short-hand such as "sounds like," "two-words," "3 words," etc." Divide the group into two or more teams with an equal number of younger and older participants on both teams. Let one member draw a game card with a song title printed on it. Next, direct the participant to provide clues to his or her team regarding the song title by using gestures. Allow 5 minutes for the team to guess the song title. The team gains 5 points if they correctly guess the song title. After guessing the song titles, play the recording for group and identify how many lyrics the participants can recall.

Level 2—Volunteer Musician

Activity Name: "Musical Jeopardy"

Advanced Preparation: Choose songs that are familiar to both generations, such as folk and patriotic songs. Also include songs that are popular with the younger participants, as well as music that is popular with the older participants, such as music from the 1930s and 1940s. Locate trivia pertaining to songs chosen for the game. Create a game board with four to five categories, and four to five answers per category. Be creative in categories, such as songs by Elvis Presley, country songs, or songs with a girl's name in the title. Answers should have a point value attached to it, such as 100, 200, etc. Create answers for all of the categories; some answers can be trivia pertaining to a song or a sound clip of the song. Create a Final Jeopardy question with a song that is familiar to both generations. Gather markers/pens and pieces of paper to use for the Final Jeopardy question.

Activity Direction: Explain the directions to the group. Divide the group into dyads consisting of one younger and one older participant. Start with group 1 and allow them to select a category and a point value. Read or play the musical clue once the category is selected. Allow each dyad 1 minute to answer the clue in a question format. The dyad receives the point value if they provide the correct question, or they lose the point value if they provide an incorrect question or are unable to provide a response. Continue among the dyads until the game board is cleared. Finish the game with the Final Jeopardy question. Direct participants to write down their questions and point values in response to the Final Jeopardy answer. The dyad with the most points wins the game.

Level 3—Board-Certified Music Therapist

Activity Name: "Getting to Know You Bingo"

Other Goals Addressed–Younger Generation: Improve Social Acceptance of Older Adults, Improve Attitudes toward Older Adults

Other Goals Addressed–Older Generation: Decrease Isolation, Improve Meaningful Interactions, Improve Attitudes toward Younger Persons

Advanced Preparation: Interview the younger and older participants to identify information about them, such as their favorite music, hobbies, families, and more. From the answers, create a bingo sheet and include items such as "find a person who has one brother," or "find a person who plays the piano." Bring enough copies of the bingo sheet and pens for each participant. Locate the chords and lyrics to the song "Getting to Know You." Provide a lyric sheet for the participants.

Activity Direction: Pass out the lyric sheets for the song to the participants. Accompany and lead the group in singing the song "Getting to Know You." After singing the song, explain the directions of the game "Getting to Know You Bingo" to the group. Pass out the bingo sheets face-side down, along with a pen. Depending on the size of the group, allow participants 10–15 minutes to complete as many bingo squares as possible. Encourage participants to interact with the other generation. Once "Getting to Know You Bingo" is complete, lead the group in a discussion of group facts. Discuss any similarities and differences between the peers and cross-age participants.

Clinical Application 4.16

Target Behavior–Younger Generation: Increase frequency of positive interactions with older adults

Target Behavior–Older Generation: Increase frequency of positive interactions with younger persons

Music: Music for this activity will be selected by the participants.

Level 1—General Staff

Activity Name: "Talent Show"

Advanced Preparation: Interview the younger and older participants to determine what talent they would like to perform in the talent show. Identify similarities among participants' responses and assign participants to groups based on their interests.

Activity Direction: When everyone in the group is present, combine individuals who have similar performance interests. Direct the groups to interview each other and identify the name of their talent and what materials they will need. Visit each group and create a list of talents and materials needed. Identify a date for the talent show and the number of rehearsals needed for groups and individuals. During rehearsals, provide assistance when needed. Before the talent show, create a program for all the participants. Invite family members and friends of the participants. Act as the MC during the talent show.

Level 2—Volunteer Musician

Activity Name: "Talent Show"

Advanced Preparation: Interview the younger and older participants to determine what talent they would like to perform in the talent show. Identify similarities among participants' responses and assign participants to groups based on their interests.

Activity Direction: When everyone in the group is present, combine individuals who have similar performance interests. Direct the groups to interview each other and identify the name of their talent and what materials they will need. Visit each group and create a list of talents and materials needed. Provide accompaniment for participants who need it on an accompaniment instrument such as guitar or piano. Identify a date for the talent show and how many rehearsals groups and individuals will have. During rehearsals, provide assistance when needed. Before the talent show, create a program for all the participants. Invite family members and friends of the participants. Act as the MC during the talent show.

Level 3—Board-Certified Music Therapist

Activity Name: "Talent Show"

Other Goals Addressed–Younger Generation: Improve Social Acceptance of Older Adults, Improve Attitudes toward Older Adults

Other Goals Addressed–Older Generation: Decrease Isolation, Improve Meaningful Interactions, Improve Attitudes toward Younger Persons

Advanced Preparation: Interview the younger and older participants to determine what talent they would like to perform in the talent show. Identify similarities among participants' responses and assign participants to groups based on their interests.

Activity Direction: When everyone in the group is present, combine individuals who have similar performance interests. Direct the groups to interview each other and identify the name of their talent and what materials they will need. Visit each group and create a list of talents and materials needed. Provide accompaniment for participants who need it on an accompaniment instrument such as guitar or piano. Teach the entire group a singing, movement, and instrument-playing act for all participants to perform at the talent show. Identify a date for the talent show and how many rehearsals groups and individuals will have. During rehearsals, provide assistance when needed. Before the talent show, create a program for all the participants. Invite family members and friends of the participants. Assign a younger and an older participant to be the MCs for the program.